Hemorrhoids

The Painful Truth About a Common Condition

Ethan D. Anderson

Xspurts.com

A New Zealand Designed Product

Other Versions Available

Why limit yourself to just one format?

This book is now available in physical, digital, and audiobook options.

Choose the way you love to read and dive into the story today. You won't regret it!

Digital ISBN: 9781776969630
Physical ISBN: 9781776969623
Audio ISBN:

To obtain a different format of this book at a discounted price, please get in touch with us at:

http://isbn.xspurts.com/

Contents

Have Questions / Comments?

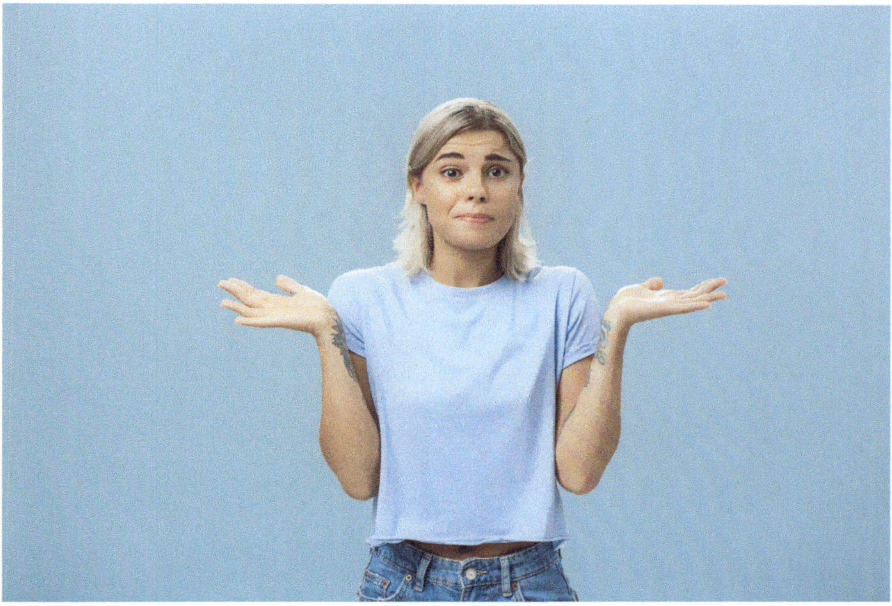

This book was designed to cover as much information as possible, but I know I have probably missed something, or some new amazing discovery has just come out.

If you notice something missing or have a question that I failed to answer, please get in touch and let me know. If I can, I will email you an answer and also update the book so others can also benefit from it.

Thanks For Being Awesome :)

Submit Your Questions / Comments At:

https://questions.xspurts.com

Get Free Stuff

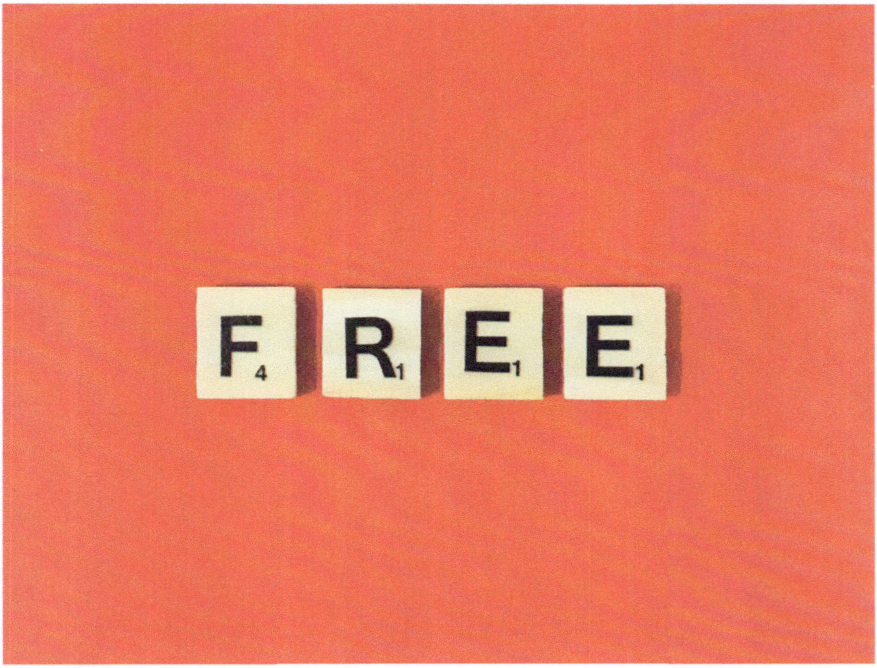

We love writing and have produced a huge number of books.

For being one of our amazing readers, we would love to offer you more books we have created, 100% free.

To claim this limited time special offer, simply go to the site below and enter your name and email address.

You will then receive loads (as we love our readers so much :) of our great books, content and audio direct to your email account, 100% free!

Get Loads of FREE Stuff at:

https://free.xspurts.com

Chapter One

Introduction

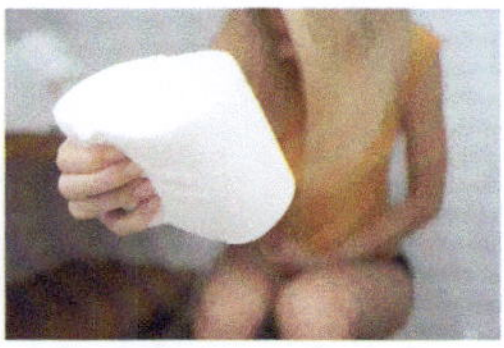

If you're reading this, then you or someone you know has hemorrhoids. And while they may not be the most pleasant topic of conversation, they are a reality for many people. In fact, it is estimated that 50% of adults will experience hemorrhoids at some point in their lives.

So what exactly are hemorrhoids? They are basically veins in the anal canal that become swollen and inflamed. There are two types of hemorrhoids: internal and external. Internal hemorrhoids are located inside the rectum and are usually not painful. External hemorrhoids, on the other hand, are located under the skin around the anus and can be painful.

There are a number of things that can cause hemorrhoids, such as pregnancy, obesity, constipation, and diarrhea. And while they can be uncomfortable, in most cases hemorrhoids are not dangerous and will go away on their own.

However, in some cases hemorrhoids can become severe and may require medical treatment. If you're dealing with hemorrhoids, this book is for you. We'll cover everything you need to know to prepare and recover from having hemorrhoids quickly and safely.

Chapter Two

What are hemorrhoids?

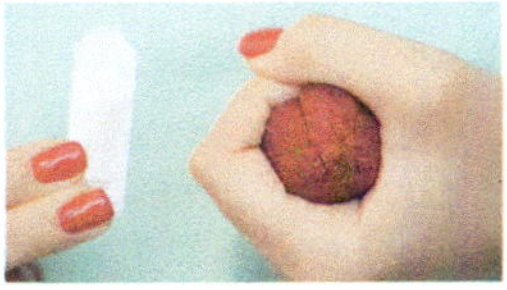

Hemorrhoids, also known as piles, are swollen veins located in the lower rectum and anus. They can be internal (inside the rectum) or external (under the skin around the anus).

The exact cause of hemorrhoids is not known, but there are several factors that can contribute to their development. One common cause is increased pressure in the lower rectum, which can be caused by constipation, diarrhea, pregnancy, or obesity. Other factors that may contribute to the development of hemorrhoids include genetics, a low-fiber diet, and a sedentary lifestyle.

Symptoms of hemorrhoids can include itching, burning, pain, and bleeding. The bleeding is usually painless and can be seen as bright red blood on toilet paper or in the toilet bowl. In some cases, a hemorrhoid can become so large that it prolapses, or protrudes, outside of the anus. This can cause discomfort and make it difficult to clean the area properly.

Hemorrhoids can be treated with a variety of methods, including lifestyle changes, over-the-counter medications, and medical procedures. Lifestyle changes, such as increasing fiber in your diet and drinking more water, can help to reduce constipation and relieve symptoms. Over-the-counter creams, ointments, and suppositories can also be used to relieve itching, burning, and pain.

If these methods are not effective, there are several medical procedures that can be used to treat hemorrhoids. One common procedure is called rubber band ligation. This involves placing a small rubber band around the base of the hemorrhoid to cut off its blood supply, causing it to shrink and eventually fall off. Another procedure is called sclerotherapy, which involves injecting a solution into the hemorrhoid to shrink it.

In severe cases, surgery may be necessary to remove the hemorrhoids. The surgery is called hemorrhoidectomy. This is typically done under general anesthesia and involves removing the hemorrhoids and the surrounding tissue. Recovery from surgery can take several weeks and may include pain, bleeding, and difficulty with bowel movements.

Hemorrhoids are a common condition that can be treated with a variety of methods. If you suspect that you have hemorrhoids, it is important to see your doctor for a proper diagnosis and treatment plan.

In order to prevent hemorrhoids from occurring, it is important to maintain a healthy diet and lifestyle. Eating a diet high in fiber, drinking plenty of water, and getting regular exercise can all help to prevent constipation and reduce the pressure in the lower rectum. Additionally, try to avoid prolonged sitting or standing, and avoid straining during bowel movements.

In conclusion, Hemorrhoids are swollen veins in the anus or lower rectum that can cause discomfort, itching, and bleeding. They can be caused by a number of factors, including constipation, diarrhea, pregnancy, and obesity. Hemorrhoids can be treated with lifestyle changes, over-the-counter medications, and medical procedures, and in severe cases, surgery may be necessary. With proper care and prevention, you can avoid the discomfort and embarrassment caused by hemorrhoids.

Definition Of Hemorrhoids

Hemorrhoids are a medical condition that occurs when the veins in the anus or rectum become swollen or inflamed. The condition is commonly referred to as piles and can be extremely uncomfortable and painful. Hemorrhoids can affect people of all ages, but are more commonly found in those over the age of 50.

1. There are two types of hemorrhoids: internal and external. Internal hemorrhoids are located inside the rectum and are generally not visible. External hemorrhoids, on the other hand, are located outside the anus and can be seen or felt as small, swollen lumps.

The exact cause of hemorrhoids is not known, but it is believed to be a combination of factors that include straining during bowel movements, constipation, prolonged sitting or standing, obesity, pregnancy, and aging. In some cases, hemorrhoids may also be caused by a family history of the condition or a medical condition that affects the veins, such as liver disease.

The symptoms of hemorrhoids can vary depending on the severity of the condition. Mild cases may only cause slight discomfort or itching, while more severe cases can cause pain, bleeding, and difficulty sitting or walking. Internal hemorrhoids may also cause bleeding during bowel movements.

The diagnosis of hemorrhoids is typically made through a physical examination of the anus and rectum. In some cases, further testing may be necessary to rule out other conditions that may be causing similar symptoms.

Treatment for hemorrhoids may include lifestyle changes, such as increasing fiber intake and exercising regularly to prevent constipation, as well as over-the-counter medications to relieve pain and itching. In some cases, prescription medications or surgery may be necessary to treat more severe cases of hemorrhoids.

Prevention of hemorrhoids can be achieved through a healthy lifestyle that includes a balanced diet, regular exercise, and good bowel habits. It is also important to avoid prolonged sitting or standing, and to maintain a healthy weight.

Hemorrhoids are a medical condition that affects the veins in the anus or rectum. The condition can cause discomfort, pain, and bleeding, and can be caused by a combination of factors such as straining during bowel movements, constipation, and obesity. Treatment for hemorrhoids may include lifestyle changes, over-the-counter medications, prescription medications, or surgery, depending on the severity of the condition. Prevention of hemorrhoids can be achieved through a healthy lifestyle that includes a balanced diet, regular exercise, and good bowel habits.

Prevalence And Demographics Of Hemorrhoids

Hemorrhoids are a common medical condition that affects millions of people around the world. The condition is more prevalent in developed countries, where the population tends to lead a sedentary lifestyle and consume a diet that is low in fiber.Below we will explore the prevalence and demographics of hemorrhoids and how they affect different populations.

According to the National Institutes of Health, approximately 50% of people over the age of 50 suffer from hemorrhoids, with the prevalence increasing with age. However, hemorrhoids can affect people of all ages, including children and teenagers. It is estimated that 4.4% of the population in the United States suffer from hemorrhoids, with men being slightly more affected than women.

The prevalence of hemorrhoids is also affected by certain demographic factors, such as race, occupation, and socioeconomic status. Studies have shown that people of African descent have a higher risk of developing hemorrhoids compared to other races. This could be due to differences in genetic predisposition, diet, or lifestyle factors.

Occupation can also play a role in the development of hemorrhoids. People who work in jobs that require prolonged sitting or standing, such as truck drivers or cashiers, have a higher risk of developing the condition. This is because prolonged sitting or standing can cause pressure on the veins in the anus or rectum, leading to inflammation and swelling.

Socioeconomic status has also been found to be a factor in the prevalence of hemorrhoids. People who live in poverty or have limited access to healthcare are more likely to develop hemorrhoids due to poor nutrition, lack of exercise, and limited access to medical treatment.

Pregnancy is another demographic factor that can increase the risk of hemorrhoids. Pregnant women experience hormonal changes that can weaken the veins in the anus or rectum, as well as increased pressure on the pelvic region due to the growing fetus. This can cause hemorrhoids to develop or worsen during pregnancy.

In terms of gender, studies have found that men are slightly more likely to develop hemorrhoids compared to women. This could be due to differences in anatomy, with men having a longer anal canal and weaker pelvic floor muscles compared to women.

The prevalence of hemorrhoids is also affected by certain health conditions. People who suffer from chronic constipation, inflammatory bowel disease, or liver disease are more likely to develop hemorrhoids. This is because these conditions can cause increased pressure on the veins in the anus or rectum, leading to inflammation and swelling.

In terms of geographic location, the prevalence of hemorrhoids is higher in developed countries compared to developing countries. This could be due to differences in lifestyle factors, such as diet and exercise, as well as access to medical treatment. Studies have found that the prevalence of hemorrhoids is highest in North America and Europe, with lower rates in Asia, Africa, and South America.

Hemorrhoids are a common medical condition that affects millions of people around the world. The prevalence of hemorrhoids is affected by demographic factors such as age, race, occupation, socioeconomic status, and gender. The condition is more prevalent in developed countries, where the population tends to lead a sedentary lifestyle and consume a diet that is low in fiber. Prevention of hemorrhoids can be achieved through a healthy lifestyle that includes a balanced diet, regular exercise, and good bowel habits. Treatment for hemorrhoids may include lifestyle changes, over-the-counter medications, prescription medications, or surgery, depending on the severity of the condition.

Myths And Misconceptions About Hemorrhoids

Hemorrhoids are a common medical condition that affect millions of people worldwide. Despite their prevalence, there are several myths and misconceptions about the condition that can make it difficult for individuals to manage the symptoms effectively. Below we will discuss some of the most common myths and misconceptions about hemorrhoids and provide accurate information to help individuals better understand the condition.

1. Myth #1: Hemorrhoids Are Caused by Sitting on Cold Surfaces

One of the most common myths about hemorrhoids is that they are caused by sitting on cold surfaces, such as concrete or metal. However, this is not true. Hemorrhoids are caused by increased pressure on the veins in the rectal and anal area, typically from straining during bowel movements, pregnancy, or obesity.

2. Myth #2: Hemorrhoids Are Contagious

Another common misconception about hemorrhoids is that they are contagious. However, hemorrhoids are not contagious and cannot be transmitted from one person to another.

3. Myth #3: Hemorrhoids Are a Sign of Poor Hygiene

Some people believe that hemorrhoids are a sign of poor hygiene, but this is not true. Hemorrhoids are caused by increased pressure on the veins in the rectal and anal area and are not related to personal hygiene.

4. Myth #4: Hemorrhoids Only Affect Older Adults

While hemorrhoids are more common in older adults, they can affect individuals of all ages. Factors such as pregnancy, obesity, and chronic constipation can increase the risk of developing hemorrhoids in younger individuals.

5. Myth #5: Hemorrhoids Always Require Surgery

Many people believe that hemorrhoids always require surgery to treat, but this is not true. In fact, most cases of hemorrhoids can be managed with self-care measures, such as increasing fiber intake, staying hydrated, and avoiding prolonged sitting.

6. Myth #6: Hemorrhoids Always Cause Pain

While hemorrhoids can cause discomfort and pain, not all cases of hemorrhoids are painful. Some individuals may experience itching, bleeding, or a feeling of fullness in the rectal area.

7. Myth #7: Hemorrhoids Are Always Visible

While external hemorrhoids are visible and can be felt as small lumps around the anus, internal hemorrhoids may not be visible. Internal hemorrhoids can cause bleeding during bowel movements and may be diagnosed during a routine physical examination.

There are several myths and misconceptions about hemorrhoids that can make it difficult for individuals to manage the condition effectively. By understanding the true causes and symptoms of hemorrhoids, individuals can better manage the condition and seek appropriate treatment when necessary. Hemorrhoids are a common medical condition that can be managed with self-care measures, medical treatments, and lifestyle changes.

Debunking Common Myths

Myths and misconceptions are often pervasive and can cause confusion, anxiety, and misunderstandings. Below we will explore some common myths and provide accurate information to debunk them.

1. Myth #1: Vaccines Cause Autism

One of the most pervasive myths in modern society is the belief that vaccines cause autism. This myth has been thoroughly debunked by numerous studies, and there is no scientific evidence to support this claim. Vaccines are safe and effective in preventing a range of illnesses, including measles, polio, and influenza.

2. Myth #2: The Earth is Flat

Despite centuries of scientific evidence, there are still individuals who believe that the Earth is flat. This myth has been thoroughly debunked by scientific evidence, including satellite imagery and global navigation technology.

3. Myth #3: Sugar Causes Hyperactivity

Many parents believe that sugar causes hyperactivity in children, but there is no scientific evidence to support this claim. While sugar can cause a temporary increase in energy, it does not cause hyperactivity or attention-deficit/hyperactivity disorder (ADHD).

4. Myth #4: You Only Use 10% of Your Brain

This popular myth suggests that humans only use 10% of their brain, leaving the remaining 90% untapped potential. However, this is not true. In reality, humans use all parts of their brain, and while certain regions may be more active during specific tasks, there is no untapped potential waiting to be unlocked.

5. Myth #5: Cracking Your Knuckles Causes Arthritis

Many people believe that cracking your knuckles can cause arthritis, but there is no scientific evidence to support this claim. While cracking your knuckles may be annoying to others, it does not cause arthritis or any other joint conditions.

6. Myth #6: A Penny Dropped from the Top of the Empire State Building Can Kill Someone

This myth suggests that dropping a penny from the top of the Empire State Building can be lethal. However, this is not true. While a penny dropped from the top of a tall building could cause injury, it would not be lethal.

7. Myth #7: Shaving Makes Hair Grow Back Thicker

This myth suggests that shaving causes hair to grow back thicker and coarser, but there is no scientific evidence to support this claim. Shaving simply cuts the hair at the surface of the skin, and the new hair that grows back is the same thickness as the previous hair.

Myths and misconceptions can be pervasive and persistent, even in the face of scientific evidence. By understanding the truth and debunking common myths, we can better understand the world around us and make informed decisions. It is important to seek out accurate information and challenge misinformation to prevent misunderstandings and promote accurate knowledge.

The Importance Of Accurate Information About Hemorrhoids

Hemorrhoids are a common medical condition that affects millions of people worldwide. However, there are many myths and misconceptions surrounding hemorrhoids that can make it difficult for individuals to manage the condition effectively. Below we will discuss the importance of accurate information about hemorrhoids and the impact it can have on individuals' health and well-being.

Accurate Information Can Help Individuals Make Informed Decisions

Accurate information about hemorrhoids can help individuals make informed decisions about how to manage the condition. This includes understanding the causes and symptoms of hemorrhoids, as well as the available treatment options. With accurate information, individuals can make choices that are best for their unique needs and circumstances.

Accurate Information Can Prevent Misdiagnosis and Mismanagement

Misinformation about hemorrhoids can lead to misdiagnosis and mismanagement of the condition. For example, individuals who believe that hemorrhoids are caused by sitting on cold surfaces may not seek the appropriate treatment for their symptoms. This can lead to further complications and prolonged suffering. Accurate information can prevent misdiagnosis and ensure that individuals receive the appropriate treatment for their condition.

Accurate Information Can Reduce Stigma and Embarrassment

Hemorrhoids are often considered a taboo subject, which can lead to feelings of embarrassment and shame for those who suffer from the condition. Accurate information about hemorrhoids can reduce stigma and help individuals feel more comfortable discussing their symptoms with healthcare providers and loved ones. This can lead to earlier diagnosis and treatment, as well as improved emotional well-being.

Accurate Information Can Improve Quality of Life

Hemorrhoids can cause significant discomfort and pain, which can impact an individual's quality of life. Accurate information about hemorrhoids can help individuals manage their symptoms effectively and improve their quality of life. This includes understanding the importance of maintaining healthy bowel habits, increasing fiber intake, and avoiding prolonged sitting.

Accurate Information Can Promote Preventative Measures

Preventing hemorrhoids can be easier than treating them. Accurate information about the causes and risk factors of hemorrhoids can help individuals take preventative measures to reduce their risk of developing the condition. This includes maintaining a healthy weight, staying hydrated, and avoiding constipation.

Accurate information about hemorrhoids is essential for individuals to manage the condition effectively and improve their quality of life. It can help prevent misdiagnosis, reduce stigma and embarrassment, promote preventative measures, and ensure that individuals receive appropriate treatment for their symptoms. Healthcare providers and individuals should work together to seek out accurate information and dispel common myths and misconceptions about hemorrhoids.

Separating Fact From Fiction

Separating fact from fiction is crucial to make informed decisions and avoid misunderstandings. In today's society, where information is easily accessible, it can be challenging to distinguish between accurate information and misinformation. Below we will explore the importance of separating fact from fiction and provide strategies for doing so.

Understand the Source of Information

One of the most important strategies for separating fact from fiction is to understand the source of information. This includes evaluating the author's credentials, checking the accuracy of the information, and determining whether the source has any biases or conflicts of interest. By understanding the source of information, individuals can determine whether the information is reliable and accurate.

Check Multiple Sources

Another strategy for separating fact from fiction is to check multiple sources. This can help individuals verify the accuracy of information and identify any discrepancies or inconsistencies. By cross-referencing information from multiple sources, individuals can gain a more comprehensive understanding of the topic and make informed decisions.

Use Evidence-Based Information

Evidence-based information is based on scientific research and clinical studies, which are conducted using rigorous methodologies and peer-reviewed by experts in the field. By using evidence-based information, individuals can rely on data-driven insights to make informed decisions.

Question Your Assumptions

Another strategy for separating fact from fiction is to question your assumptions. This includes challenging preconceived notions and biases that may affect your perception of the information. By questioning your assumptions, you can approach the information with an open mind and evaluate it objectively.

Consult with Experts

Consulting with experts is another effective strategy for separating fact from fiction. Experts in the field can provide valuable insights and perspectives on complex topics, and can help individuals make informed decisions. By consulting with experts, individuals can gain a deeper understanding of the topic and avoid misinformation.

Separating fact from fiction is crucial in today's information age. By understanding the source of information, checking multiple sources, using evidence-based information, questioning assumptions, and consulting with experts, individuals can make informed decisions and avoid misunderstandings. It is essential to seek out accurate information and challenge misinformation to promote accurate knowledge and prevent misunderstandings. By doing so, individuals can make informed decisions and contribute to a more informed and engaged society.

The Anatomy Of Hemorrhoids

Hemorrhoids are a medical condition that affects the veins in the anus or rectum, causing them to become swollen and inflamed. In order to understand how hemorrhoids develop and how they are treated, it is important to have a basic understanding of the anatomy of the anus and rectum.

The anus and rectum are part of the digestive system, which is responsible for processing and eliminating waste from the body. The anus is the opening at the end of the digestive tract, through which fecal matter is expelled from the body. The rectum is the final section of the large intestine, where fecal matter is stored until it is ready to be eliminated.

1. The veins in the anus and rectum are an important part of the anatomy, as they are responsible for draining blood from the area. These veins are called hemorrhoidal veins, and they are located in two main areas: the internal hemorrhoidal plexus and the external hemorrhoidal plexus.

The internal hemorrhoidal plexus is located in the upper part of the anal canal, above the internal anal sphincter. These veins are not visible from the outside and are covered by a layer of mucous membrane. When these veins become swollen or inflamed, they can cause internal hemorrhoids, which are not visible but can cause discomfort or bleeding during bowel movements.

The external hemorrhoidal plexus is located in the lower part of the anal canal, below the internal anal sphincter. These veins are visible from the outside and are covered by a layer of skin. When these veins become swollen or inflamed, they can cause external hemorrhoids, which are visible as small, swollen lumps around the anus.

The internal and external hemorrhoidal plexus are connected by small veins called bridging veins. These veins allow blood to flow between the two plexuses, and can also become swollen or inflamed, causing discomfort or bleeding.

The anatomy of the anus and rectum also includes several muscles that are responsible for controlling bowel movements. The internal anal sphincter is a smooth muscle that is controlled by the autonomic nervous system, and is responsible for keeping the anus closed. The external anal sphincter is a skeletal muscle that is under conscious control, and is responsible for allowing bowel movements to occur.

When hemorrhoids develop, it is often due to increased pressure on the hemorrhoidal veins in the anus or rectum. This increased pressure can be caused by a variety of factors, such as constipation, straining during bowel movements, pregnancy, or obesity. When the veins become swollen or inflamed, they can cause discomfort, pain, bleeding, or itching.

Treatment for hemorrhoids typically involves lifestyle changes, such as increasing fiber intake and exercising regularly to prevent constipation, as well as over-the-counter medications to relieve pain and itching. In some cases, prescription medications or surgery may be necessary to treat more severe cases of hemorrhoids.

The Rectal And Anal Area

The rectal and anal area is an important part of the human anatomy, as it is responsible for the elimination of waste from the body. This area is composed of several different structures, including the anus, rectum, and surrounding muscles and tissues. Understanding the anatomy of the rectal and anal area can help individuals better understand how this area functions, and can also help healthcare providers diagnose and treat various medical conditions that affect this area.

1. The anus is the opening at the end of the digestive tract through which fecal matter is eliminated from the body. The anus is composed of two main parts: the internal anal sphincter and the external anal sphincter.

The internal anal sphincter is a smooth muscle that is controlled by the autonomic nervous system and is responsible for keeping the anus closed. The external anal sphincter is a skeletal muscle that is under conscious control and is responsible for allowing bowel movements to occur.

The rectum is the final section of the large intestine, where fecal matter is stored until it is ready to be eliminated. The rectum is composed of several layers of muscles and tissues, including the rectal mucosa, submucosa, and muscularis externa. These layers work together to help move fecal matter through the rectum and out of the body.

The anal canal is the section of the rectum that leads to the anus. The anal canal is composed of several layers of muscles and tissues, including the internal anal sphincter, external anal sphincter, and the anal cushions. The anal cushions are small pads of tissue that help to seal the anal canal, preventing the leakage of fecal matter.

2. The anal canal is also home to the hemorrhoidal veins, which are responsible for draining blood from the area. These veins are located in two main areas: the internal hemorrhoidal plexus and the external hemorrhoidal plexus. The internal hemorrhoidal plexus is located in the upper part of the anal canal, above the internal anal sphincter. These veins are not visible from the outside and are covered by a layer of mucous membrane. When these veins become swollen or inflamed, they can cause internal hemorrhoids, which are not visible but can cause discomfort or bleeding during bowel movements. The external hemorrhoidal plexus is located in the lower part of the anal canal, below the internal anal sphincter. These veins are visible from the outside and are covered by a layer of skin. When these veins become swollen or inflamed, they can cause external hemorrhoids, which are visible as small, swollen lumps around the anus.

The anal and rectal area is also home to several types of glands, including the anal glands and the rectal glands. These glands produce mucus, which helps to lubricate the anal canal and facilitate the passage of fecal matter. The anal glands are located just inside the anus, while the rectal glands are located in the lining of the rectum.

The anatomy of the anal and rectal area is important in understanding the various medical conditions that can affect this area. For example, hemorrhoids are a common condition that occurs when the veins in the anal and rectal area become swollen or inflamed. Other conditions that can affect this area include anal fissures, abscesses, and fistulas.

Internal And External Hemorrhoids

1. Hemorrhoids are a medical condition that affects the veins in the anus or rectum, causing them to become swollen and inflamed. There are two types of hemorrhoids: internal hemorrhoids and external hemorrhoids.B elow we will explore the differences between internal and external hemorrhoids, their symptoms, and how they are treated.

Internal hemorrhoids are located in the upper part of the anal canal, above the internal anal sphincter. These veins are not visible from the outside and are covered by a layer of mucous membrane. When these veins become swollen or inflamed, they can cause internal hemorrhoids. Internal hemorrhoids can be classified into four grades, depending on the severity of the condition.

Grade 1 internal hemorrhoids are small, and usually do not cause any symptoms. They may bleed during bowel movements, but otherwise do not cause discomfort or pain.

Grade 2 internal hemorrhoids are larger and may protrude outside of the anus during bowel movements. They may cause discomfort, itching, or bleeding during bowel movements.

Grade 3 internal hemorrhoids are even larger and may protrude outside of the anus during bowel movements, but usually retract back inside on their own. They may cause pain, bleeding, or discomfort during bowel movements.

Grade 4 internal hemorrhoids are the most severe, and cannot be pushed back inside the anus. They may cause constant pain, bleeding, and discomfort, and may require surgery to treat.

2. External hemorrhoids are located in the lower part of the anal canal, below the internal anal sphincter. These veins are visible from the outside and are covered by a layer of skin. When these veins become swollen or inflamed, they can cause external hemorrhoids. External hemorrhoids can be classified into two types: acute and chronic.

Acute external hemorrhoids are typically caused by a blood clot in the veins, and can cause severe pain, itching, or discomfort. They may also appear as a small, swollen lump around the anus. Acute external hemorrhoids usually resolve on their own within a few days, but may require treatment to relieve symptoms.

Chronic external hemorrhoids are a more long-term condition, and may cause discomfort, itching, or bleeding during bowel movements. They may also appear as small, swollen lumps around the anus. Chronic external hemorrhoids can be treated with lifestyle changes, such as increasing fiber intake and exercising regularly to prevent constipation, as well as over-the-counter medications to relieve pain and itching. In some cases, prescription medications or surgery may be necessary to treat more severe cases of hemorrhoids.

Hemorrhoidal Veins And Their Function

1. The hemorrhoidal veins are an important part of the anatomy of the anus and rectum. These veins are responsible for draining blood from the area, and are located in two main areas: the internal hemorrhoidal plexus and the external hemorrhoidal plexus.

The internal hemorrhoidal plexus is located in the upper part of the anal canal, above the internal anal sphincter. These veins are not visible from the outside and are covered by a layer of mucous membrane. The internal hemorrhoidal plexus is responsible for draining blood from the rectum and anus, and plays an important role in the process of defecation.

The external hemorrhoidal plexus is located in the lower part of the anal canal, below the internal anal sphincter. These veins are visible from the outside and are covered by a layer of skin. The external hemorrhoidal plexus is responsible for draining blood from the skin around the anus, and plays a role in the body's immune system by helping to fight off infections.

The hemorrhoidal veins are important because they help to regulate blood flow in the anus and rectum. When the veins become swollen or inflamed, they can cause hemorrhoids, which can be painful and uncomfortable. Hemorrhoids can be caused by a variety of factors, including constipation, straining during bowel movements, pregnancy, or obesity.

Treatment for hemorrhoids typically involves lifestyle changes, such as increasing fiber intake and exercising regularly to prevent constipation, as well as over-the-counter medications to relieve pain and itching. In some cases, prescription medications or surgery may be necessary to treat more severe cases of hemorrhoids.

It is important to note that the hemorrhoidal veins can also be affected by other medical conditions, such as anal fissures, abscesses, or fistulas. These conditions can cause similar symptoms to hemorrhoids, such as pain, itching, or bleeding during bowel movements, and may require different treatment approaches.

In addition to their role in regulating blood flow, the hemorrhoidal veins also play a role in the immune system. The veins are surrounded by a network of lymphatic vessels, which help to remove waste and toxins from the area. This lymphatic system plays an important role in the body's immune system, as it helps to remove harmful substances from the body and prevent infections.

Chapter Three

How do you get hemorrhoids

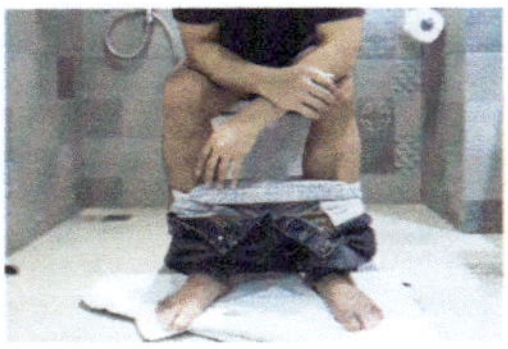

Hemorrhoids, also known as piles, are swollen veins in the lower rectum and anus. They can be caused by a variety of factors, including constipation, diarrhea, and straining during bowel movements.

One of the main causes of hemorrhoids is increased pressure in the lower rectal area. This pressure can be caused by a variety of factors, including constipation. When stools become hard and difficult to pass, it can put extra strain on the veins in the rectum and anus, causing them to become swollen and inflamed.

Another common cause of hemorrhoids is diarrhea. When stools are loose and watery, it can also put extra pressure on the veins in the rectal area, causing them to become swollen and inflamed.

Straining during bowel movements can also cause hemorrhoids. When you strain to push out a bowel movement, it can put extra pressure on the veins in the rectal area, causing them to become swollen and inflamed. This is why hemorrhoids are often more common in people who have trouble with constipation or who have to strain to have a bowel movement.

Obesity and pregnancy can also increase the risk of developing hemorrhoids. Being overweight can put extra pressure on the veins in the rectal area, and pregnancy can cause hormonal changes that can lead to hemorrhoids.

Sitting for long periods of time can also increase the risk of developing hemorrhoids, as it can cause the veins in the rectal area to become compressed. This is why hemorrhoids are often more common in people who have sedentary jobs or who spend a lot of time sitting.

Hemorrhoids can also be caused by certain medical conditions, such as Crohn's disease and diverticulitis. These conditions can cause inflammation in the rectal area, which can lead to hemorrhoids.

Symptoms of hemorrhoids include itching, pain, and bleeding during bowel movements. In some cases, hemorrhoids can also cause a lump to form around the anus, which can be painful and itchy.

If you have hemorrhoids, there are a number of things you can do to help relieve symptoms and prevent them from getting worse. For example, you can try to keep your stools soft by eating a diet that is high in fiber and drinking plenty of water. You can also try to avoid straining during bowel movements, as this can put extra pressure on the veins in the rectal area.

If you're experiencing hemorrhoids, it's also important to take steps to avoid constipation, as hard stools can put extra pressure on the veins in the rectal area. Eating a diet that is high in fiber and drinking plenty of water can help prevent constipation and keep stools soft.

If you're experiencing hemorrhoids, you may also want to consider using over-the-counter creams or ointments to help relieve symptoms. These creams and ointments can help to reduce inflammation and itching, and may also help to shrink the hemorrhoids.

In severe cases, surgery may be required to remove the hemorrhoids. Surgery is typically only recommended if other treatments are not successful, and if the hemorrhoids are causing severe pain or bleeding.

In conclusion, Hemorrhoids are caused by increased pressure in the lower rectal area, which can be caused by a variety of factors, including constipation, diarrhea, straining during bowel movements, obesity and pregnancy, sitting for long periods of time, and certain medical conditions. Symptoms include itching, pain, and bleeding during bowel movements.

Chapter Four

What are the symptoms of hemorrhoids

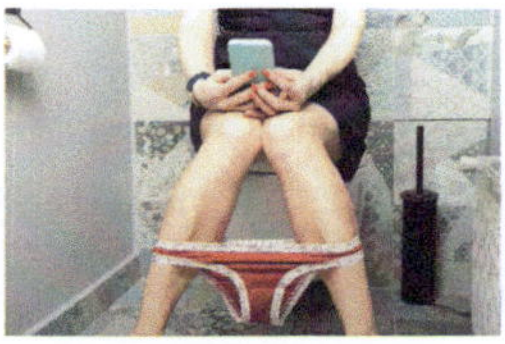

Hemorrhoids, also known as piles, are swollen veins located in the lower rectum and anus. They can be internal, meaning they are inside the rectum, or external, meaning they are outside the anus.

The most common symptom of hemorrhoids is painless bleeding during bowel movements. You may notice small amounts of bright red blood on toilet paper or in the toilet bowl. Other symptoms include itching, discomfort or pain in the rectal area, and a feeling of fullness in the rectum.

In the case of external hemorrhoids, you may also experience a lump or swelling around the anus. This can be accompanied by pain, especially when sitting or during bowel movements. In some cases, the hemorrhoid may even prolapse, or bulge out of the anus.

Internal hemorrhoids, on the other hand, are generally not visible and may not cause any symptoms at all. However, if they become enlarged, they can cause rectal bleeding, discomfort, and itching.

Hemorrhoids can also be accompanied by other symptoms such as constipation, diarrhea, and straining during bowel movements. These symptoms can exacerbate the condition, making it even more uncomfortable.

There are also different grades of hemorrhoids, with grade 1 being the mildest and grade 4 being the most severe. Grade 1 hemorrhoids are usually not visible and cause minimal symptoms, while grade 4 hemorrhoids are enlarged and prolapsed, making them visible outside the anus and causing severe discomfort and pain.

In some cases, hemorrhoids can become thrombosed, meaning a blood clot has formed in the vein. This can cause severe pain and swelling, and may require immediate medical attention.

While hemorrhoids are a common condition, it is important to note that rectal bleeding can also be a symptom of other serious conditions, such as colorectal cancer. If you experience rectal bleeding or other symptoms of hemorrhoids, it is important to see a doctor to rule out any underlying conditions.

There are a number of treatment options available for hemorrhoids, depending on the severity of the condition. These can include over-the-counter creams and ointments, home remedies such as sitz baths and witch hazel, and in more severe cases, surgery.

In general, it is important to maintain a healthy diet and lifestyle to prevent the development of hemorrhoids. This can include eating a high-fiber diet, staying hydrated, and getting regular exercise. It is also important to avoid straining during bowel movements and to practice good hygiene to keep the area clean and reduce the risk of infection.

In conclusion, hemorrhoids are a common condition that can cause symptoms such as rectal bleeding, itching, discomfort and pain. Symptoms can vary depending on whether the hemorrhoids are internal or external, and can be accompanied by other symptoms such as constipation, diarrhea, and straining during bowel movements.

Chapter Five

What causes hemorrhoids?

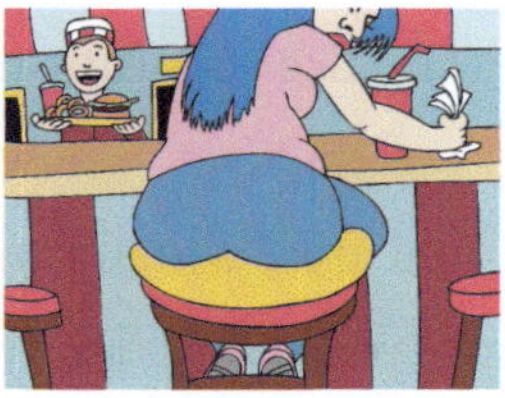

Hemorrhoids, also known as piles, are a common condition that affects the veins in the lower rectum and anus. They can be a painful and embarrassing problem, but the good news is that they are usually not serious and can often be treated at home. In this chapter, we'll explore the causes of hemorrhoids in detail, so you can understand what's going on in your body and how to best treat them.

One of the most common causes of hemorrhoids is chronic constipation. When you're constipated, you may strain to have a bowel movement, which can put pressure on the veins in your rectum and anus. This can cause the veins to become swollen and inflamed, leading to hemorrhoids. Additionally, if you're frequently having hard stools, it can also cause trauma to the rectal and anal area, which again can lead to hemorrhoids.

Another common cause of hemorrhoids is pregnancy. During pregnancy, the growing uterus puts pressure on the veins in the pelvic area, which can cause the veins in the rectum and anus to become swollen and inflamed. Additionally, hormonal changes during pregnancy can cause the veins to relax and expand, further exacerbating the problem.

Other factors that can contribute to the development of hemorrhoids include obesity, a sedentary lifestyle, and a diet that is high in processed foods and low in fiber. Obesity can put extra pressure on the veins in the rectum and anus, while a sedentary lifestyle can lead to a lack of muscle tone in the area, making it more difficult to have a bowel movement. A diet that is low in fiber can also contribute to constipation, which can further exacerbate the problem.

In some cases, hemorrhoids can also be caused by a medical condition such as inflammatory bowel disease (IBD) or cirrhosis of the liver. These conditions can cause inflammation in the rectal and anal area, which can lead to the development of hemorrhoids. Additionally, if you have a family history of hemorrhoids, you may be more likely to develop them yourself.

So, there you have it – an in-depth look at the causes of hemorrhoids. As you can see, there are a variety of factors that can contribute to the development of this condition, and understanding the underlying cause can help you determine the best course of treatment. If you suspect you have hemorrhoids, it's always a good idea to speak with your healthcare provider, who can help diagnose the problem and recommend treatment options.

In the meantime, there are a few things you can do to help alleviate symptoms and prevent hemorrhoids from becoming worse. Eating a diet high in fiber and drinking plenty of water can help prevent constipation and reduce the pressure on the veins in your rectum and anus. Additionally, regular exercise can help improve muscle tone in the area, making it easier to have a bowel movement.

If you already have hemorrhoids, there are a number of treatments available to help alleviate symptoms and reduce inflammation. Over-the-counter creams and ointments can provide temporary relief, while certain home remedies, such as soaking in a warm bath or using a cold compress, can also be helpful. In severe cases, your healthcare provider may recommend more invasive treatments such as rubber band ligation or surgery.

In conclusion, hemorrhoids are a common condition that affects many people, and understanding the underlying causes can help you determine the best course of treatment. If you suspect you have hemorrhoids, speak with your healthcare provider, who can help diagnose the problem and recommend treatment options.

Causes Of Hemorrhoids: Straining During Bowel Movements

Hemorrhoids are a common medical condition that affects millions of people worldwide. There are several factors that can contribute to the development of hemorrhoids, one of which is straining during bowel mov ements.Below we will explore the causes of hemorrhoids and how straining during bowel movements can lead to their development.

Hemorrhoids are caused by increased pressure on the veins in the anus or rectum. This increased pressure can be caused by a variety of factors, including:

1. Constipation: Constipation is a common cause of hemorrhoids, as it can cause the stool to become hard and difficult to pass. This can lead to straining during bowel movements, which can increase the pressure on the veins in the anus or rectum.

2. Diarrhea: Diarrhea can also contribute to the development of hemorrhoids, as it can cause frequent bowel movements and increase the pressure on the veins in the anus or rectum.

3. Pregnancy: Pregnancy is another common cause of hemorrhoids, as the growing fetus can put pressure on the veins in the pelvic area, leading to the development of hemorrhoids.

4. Obesity: Being overweight or obese can also contribute to the development of hemorrhoids, as the excess weight can put pressure on the veins in the anus or rectum.

5. Sitting or standing for long periods: Sitting or standing for long periods can also increase the pressure on the veins in the anus or rectum, leading to the development of hemorrhoids.

One of the most common causes of hemorrhoids is straining during bowel movements. Straining can occur when the stool is hard and difficult to pass, and can increase the pressure on the veins in the anus or rectum. Straining can be caused by several factors, including:

6. Lack of fiber: A lack of fiber in the diet can lead to constipation, which can cause the stool to become hard and difficult to pass, leading to straining during bowel movements.

7. Dehydration: Dehydration can also contribute to the development of constipation and straining during bowel movements.

8. Ignoring the urge to defecate: Ignoring the urge to defecate can lead to constipation and straining during bowel movements, as the stool can become harder and more difficult to pass the longer it stays in the colon.

9. Medical conditions: Certain medical conditions, such as irritable bowel syndrome (IBS) or inflammatory bowel disease (IBD), can also contribute to the development of constipation and straining during bowel movements.

Straining during bowel movements can cause the veins in the anus or rectum to become swollen and inflamed, leading to the development of hemorrhoids. Symptoms of hemorrhoids can include pain, itching, bleeding, and discomfort during bowel movements. Treatment for hemorrhoids typically involves lifestyle changes, such as increasing fiber intake and exercising regularly to prevent constipation, as well as over-the-counter medications to relieve pain and itching. In some cases, prescription medications or surgery may be necessary to treat more severe cases of hemorrhoids.

Causes Of Hemorrhoids: Prolonged Sitting

Hemorrhoids are a common medical condition that affects millions of people worldwide. There are several factors that can contribute to the development of hemorrhoids, one of which is prolonged sitting.Below we will explore the causes of hemorrhoids and how prolonged sitting can lead to their development.

Hemorrhoids are caused by increased pressure on the veins in the anus or rectum. This increased pressure can be caused by a variety of factors, including:

1. Constipation: Constipation is a common cause of hemorrhoids, as it can cause the stool to become hard and difficult to pass. This can lead to straining during bowel movements, which can increase the pressure on the veins in the anus or rectum.

2. Diarrhea: Diarrhea can also contribute to the development of hemorrhoids, as it can cause frequent bowel movements and increase the pressure on the veins in the anus or rectum.

3. Pregnancy: Pregnancy is another common cause of hemorrhoids, as the growing fetus can put pressure on the veins in the pelvic area, leading to the development of hemorrhoids.

4. Obesity: Being overweight or obese can also contribute to the development of hemorrhoids, as the excess weight can put pressure on the veins in the anus or rectum.

5. Straining during bowel movements: Straining during bowel movements can also increase the pressure on the veins in the anus or rectum, leading to the development of hemorrhoids.

One of the lesser-known causes of hemorrhoids is prolonged sitting. Prolonged sitting can lead to the development of hemorrhoids by increasing the pressure on the veins in the anus or rectum. This increased pressure can be caused by several factors, including:

6. Sitting for long periods: Sitting for long periods can increase the pressure on the veins in the anus or rectum, especially if the seat is hard or uncomfortable.

7. Sitting with poor posture: Sitting with poor posture can also contribute to the development of hemorrhoids, as it can increase the pressure on the veins in the anus or rectum.

8. Sitting on a toilet for too long: Sitting on a toilet for too long can also increase the pressure on the veins in the anus or rectum, especially if the toilet seat is hard or uncomfortable.

Prolonged sitting can cause the veins in the anus or rectum to become swollen and inflamed, leading to the development of hemorrhoids. Symptoms of hemorrhoids can include pain, itching, bleeding, and discomfort during bowel movements. Treatment for hemorrhoids typically involves lifestyle changes, such as increasing fiber intake and exercising regularly to prevent constipation, as well as over-the-counter medications to relieve pain and itching. In some cases, prescription medications or surgery may be necessary to treat more severe cases of hemorrhoids.

To prevent the development of hemorrhoids from prolonged sitting, it is important to take breaks from sitting regularly. This can be achieved by standing up and stretching, taking a short walk, or performing simple exercises. It is also important to maintain good posture while sitting, and to use a comfortable and supportive seat.

Causes Of Hemorrhoids: Pregnancy And Childbirth

Pregnancy and childbirth are major life events that can have a significant impact on a woman's body. One common issue that can arise during pregnancy and childbirth is hemorrhoids.Below we will explore the causes of hemorrhoids during pregnancy and childbirth, as well as their symptoms and treatment options.

Hemorrhoids are caused by increased pressure on the veins in the anus or rectum. During pregnancy, the growing fetus puts pressure on the pelvic area, which can lead to increased pressure on the veins in the anus or rectum. Additionally, hormonal changes during pregnancy can cause the walls of the veins to relax, making them more susceptible to swelling and inflammation.

During childbirth, the pushing and straining that occurs during labor can also increase the pressure on the veins in the anus or rectum, leading to the development of hemorrhoids. Additionally, the use of forceps or other instruments during delivery can increase the risk of developing hemorrhoids.

Symptoms of hemorrhoids during pregnancy and childbirth can include pain, itching, bleeding, and discomfort during bowel movements. Treatment for hemorrhoids during pregnancy and childbirth typically involves lifestyle changes, such as increasing fiber intake and exercising regularly to prevent constipation, as well as over-the-counter medications to relieve pain and itching. In some cases, prescription medications or surgery may be necessary to treat more severe cases of hemorrhoids.

Preventing hemorrhoids during pregnancy and childbirth can be achieved by taking certain precautions, such as:

1. Eating a healthy, high-fiber diet: A diet rich in fiber can help to prevent constipation and straining during bowel movements, which can lead to the development of hemorrhoids.

2. Staying hydrated: Drinking plenty of water can help to prevent constipation and keep the stools soft and easy to pass.

3. Exercising regularly: Regular exercise can help to improve circulation and prevent constipation.

4. Taking breaks from sitting or standing for long periods: Taking breaks from sitting or standing for long periods can help to reduce pressure on the veins in the anus or rectum.

5. Using a donut-shaped pillow: Using a donut-shaped pillow while sitting can help to reduce pressure on the veins in the anus or rectum.

Causes Of Hemorrhoids: Obesity

Hemorrhoids are a common medical condition that affects millions of people worldwide. There are several factors that can contribute to the development of hemorrhoids, one of which is obesity.Below we will explore the causes of hemorrhoids and how obesity can lead to their development.

Hemorrhoids are caused by increased pressure on the veins in the anus or rectum. This increased pressure can be caused by a variety of factors, including:

1. Constipation: Constipation is a common cause of hemorrhoids, as it can cause the stool to become hard and difficult to pass. This can lead to straining during bowel movements, which can increase the pressure on the veins in the anus or rectum.

2. Diarrhea: Diarrhea can also contribute to the development of hemorrhoids, as it can cause frequent bowel movements and increase the pressure on the veins in the anus or rectum.

3. Pregnancy: Pregnancy is another common cause of hemorrhoids, as the growing fetus can put pressure on the veins in the pelvic area, leading to the development of hemorrhoids.

4. Prolonged sitting: Sitting for long periods can also increase the pressure on the veins in the anus or rectum, leading to the development of hemorrhoids.

5. Obesity: Being overweight or obese can also contribute to the development of hemorrhoids, as the excess weight can put pressure on the veins in the anus or rectum.

Obesity is a major risk factor for the development of hemorrhoids. Excess weight can put pressure on the veins in the anus or rectum, leading to the development of hemorrhoids. Additionally, obesity can contribute to constipation, which can cause straining during bowel movements and increase the pressure on the veins in the anus or rectum.

Symptoms of hemorrhoids can include pain, itching, bleeding, and discomfort during bowel movements. Treatment for hemorrhoids typically involves lifestyle changes, such as increasing fiber intake and exercising regularly to prevent constipation, as well as over-the-counter medications to relieve pain and itching. In some cases, prescription medications or surgery may be necessary to treat more severe cases of hemorrhoids.

To prevent the development of hemorrhoids from obesity, it is important to maintain a healthy weight through diet and exercise. Eating a healthy, balanced diet that is rich in fiber can help to prevent constipation and reduce the risk of developing hemorrhoids. Regular exercise can also help to improve circulation and prevent constipation.

Causes Of Hemorrhoids: Chronic Constipation Or Diarrhea

Hemorrhoids are a common medical condition that affects millions of people worldwide. There are several factors that can contribute to the development of hemorrhoids, one of which is chronic constipation or diarrhea.Below we will explore the causes of hemorrhoids and how chronic constipation or diarrhea can lead to their development.

Hemorrhoids are caused by increased pressure on the veins in the anus or rectum. This increased pressure can be caused by a variety of factors, including:

1. Constipation: Constipation is a common cause of hemorrhoids, as it can cause the stool to become hard and difficult to pass. This can lead to straining during bowel movements, which can increase the pressure on the veins in the anus or rectum.

2. Diarrhea: Diarrhea can also contribute to the development of hemorrhoids, as it can cause frequent bowel movements and increase the pressure on the veins in the anus or rectum.

3. Pregnancy: Pregnancy is another common cause of hemorrhoids, as the growing fetus can put pressure on the veins in the pelvic area, leading to the development of hemorrhoids.

4. Prolonged sitting: Sitting for long periods can also increase the pressure on the veins in the anus or rectum, leading to the development of hemorrhoids.

5. Obesity: Being overweight or obese can also contribute to the development of hemorrhoids, as the excess weight can put pressure on the veins in the anus or rectum.

Chronic constipation or diarrhea can lead to the development of hemorrhoids. Constipation can cause the stool to become hard and difficult to pass, leading to straining during bowel movements and increased pressure on the veins in the anus or rectum. Chronic diarrhea can cause frequent bowel movements and increased pressure on the veins in the anus or rectum, leading to the development of hemorrhoids.

Symptoms of hemorrhoids can include pain, itching, bleeding, and discomfort during bowel movements. Treatment for hemorrhoids typically involves lifestyle changes, such as increasing fiber intake and exercising regularly to prevent constipation, as well as over-the-counter medications to relieve pain and itching. In some cases, prescription medications or surgery may be necessary to treat more severe cases of hemorrhoids.

To prevent the development of hemorrhoids from chronic constipation or diarrhea, it is important to maintain a healthy diet and exercise regularly. A diet that is rich in fiber can help to prevent constipation and reduce the risk of developing hemorrhoids. Regular exercise can also help to improve circulation and prevent constipation.

Causes Of Hemorrhoids: Aging

Hemorrhoids are a common medical condition that affects millions of people worldwide. There are several factors that can contribute to the development of hemorrhoids, one of which is aging.Below we will explore the causes of hemorrhoids and how aging can lead to their development.

Hemorrhoids are caused by increased pressure on the veins in the anus or rectum. This increased pressure can be caused by a variety of factors, including:

1. Constipation: Constipation is a common cause of hemorrhoids, as it can cause the stool to become hard and difficult to pass. This can lead to straining during bowel movements, which can increase the pressure on the veins in the anus or rectum.

2. Diarrhea: Diarrhea can also contribute to the development of hemorrhoids, as it can cause frequent bowel movements and increase the pressure on the veins in the anus or rectum.

3. Pregnancy: Pregnancy is another common cause of hemorrhoids, as the growing fetus can put pressure on the veins in the pelvic area, leading to the development of hemorrhoids.

4. Prolonged sitting: Sitting for long periods can also increase the pressure on the veins in the anus or rectum, leading to the development of hemorrhoids.

5. Obesity: Being overweight or obese can also contribute to the development of hemorrhoids, as the excess weight can put pressure on the veins in the anus or rectum.

As people age, the risk of developing hemorrhoids increases. This is because the tissues and muscles in the anus and rectum can weaken with age, making them more susceptible to swelling and inflammation. Additionally, aging can lead to other factors that can contribute to the development of hemorrhoids, such as constipation and prolonged sitting.

Symptoms of hemorrhoids can include pain, itching, bleeding, and discomfort during bowel movements. Treatment for hemorrhoids typically involves lifestyle changes, such as increasing fiber intake and exercising regularly to prevent constipation, as well as over-the-counter medications to relieve pain and itching. In some cases, prescription medications or surgery may be necessary to treat more severe cases of hemorrhoids.

To prevent the development of hemorrhoids from aging, it is important to maintain a healthy diet and exercise regularly. A diet that is rich in fiber can help to prevent constipation and reduce the risk of developing hemorrhoids. Regular exercise can also help to improve circulation and prevent constipation.

Causes Of Hemorrhoids: Genetics

Hemorrhoids are a common medical condition that affects millions of people worldwide. There are several factors that can contribute to the development of hemorrhoids, one of which is genetics.Below we will explore the causes of hemorrhoids and how genetics can lead to their development.

Hemorrhoids are caused by increased pressure on the veins in the anus or rectum. This increased pressure can be caused by a variety of factors, including:

1. Constipation: Constipation is a common cause of hemorrhoids, as it can cause the stool to become hard and difficult to pass. This can lead to straining during bowel movements, which can increase the pressure on the veins in the anus or rectum.

2. Diarrhea: Diarrhea can also contribute to the development of hemorrhoids, as it can cause frequent bowel movements and increase the pressure on the veins in the anus or rectum.

3. Pregnancy: Pregnancy is another common cause of hemorrhoids, as the growing fetus can put pressure on the veins in the pelvic area, leading to the development of hemorrhoids.

4. Prolonged sitting: Sitting for long periods can also increase the pressure on the veins in the anus or rectum, leading to the development of hemorrhoids.

5. Obesity: Being overweight or obese can also contribute to the development of hemorrhoids, as the excess weight can put pressure on the veins in the anus or rectum.

Genetics can also play a role in the development of hemorrhoids. Studies have shown that there may be a genetic predisposition to the development of hemorrhoids, with certain genes being associated with an increased risk of developing the condition. Additionally, some inherited conditions, such as Ehlers-Danlos syndrome, can increase the risk of developing hemorrhoids.

Symptoms of hemorrhoids can include pain, itching, bleeding, and discomfort during bowel movements. Treatment for hemorrhoids typically involves lifestyle changes, such as increasing fiber intake and exercising regularly to prevent constipation, as well as over-the-counter medications to relieve pain and itching. In some cases, prescription medications or surgery may be necessary to treat more severe cases of hemorrhoids.

To prevent the development of hemorrhoids from genetics, it is important to maintain a healthy lifestyle and discuss any family history of hemorrhoids or related conditions with a healthcare provider. Eating a diet that is rich in fiber can help to prevent constipation and reduce the risk of developing hemorrhoids. Regular exercise can also help to improve circulation and prevent constipation.

Chapter Six

Internal hemorrhoids

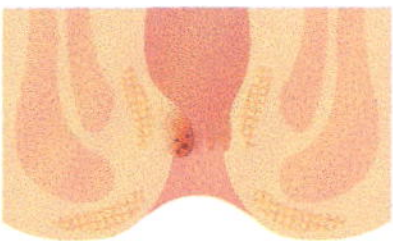

Internal hemorrhoids are a common condition that affects the veins in the lower rectum and anus. They are caused by increased pressure on the veins in these areas, which can be due to a variety of factors such as constipation, diarrhea, pregnancy, genetics, and even prolonged sitting or standing.

Symptoms of internal hemorrhoids can include rectal bleeding, itching, and pain. The bleeding is usually painless and can be seen on toilet paper or in the toilet bowl after a bowel movement. Itching and discomfort may also occur, but this is not always the case. Some people may have internal hemorrhoids and not experience any symptoms at all.

There are several different stages of internal hemorrhoids, each with its own set of symptoms. The first stage is characterized by small, swollen veins in the anus or rectum that may be itchy or bleed slightly. In the second stage, the veins become larger and more swollen, and can prolapse, or bulge out of the anus. In the third stage, the hemorrhoids hang out of the anus and must be manually pushed back in after a bowel movement. The fourth and most severe stage is characterized by hemorrhoids that are permanently prolapsed and cannot be pushed back into the anus.

Treatment for internal hemorrhoids depends on the stage and severity of the condition. For mild cases, changes in diet and bowel habits can be enough to alleviate symptoms. Eating a high-fiber diet, drinking plenty of water, and engaging in regular exercise can help to prevent constipation and reduce pressure on the veins in the anus and rectum. Over-the-counter creams and ointments can also be used to relieve itching and discomfort.

For more severe cases, there are several different options available. Rubber band ligation is a common procedure in which a small rubber band is placed around the base of the hemorrhoid, cutting off its blood supply and causing it to shrink and fall off. Sclerotherapy is another option that involves injecting a solution into the hemorrhoid to shrink it. Hemorrhoidectomy is a surgical procedure that involves the removal of the hemorrhoid.

In addition, there are some natural remedies that can help to alleviate symptoms of internal hemorrhoids and may be worth trying before moving on to more invasive treatments. Witch hazel, for example, can be applied topically to reduce itching and pain. Aloe vera gel can also be used to soothe the area and reduce inflammation.

Internal hemorrhoids can be a very uncomfortable condition, but there are many effective treatment options available. With the right diet and lifestyle changes, as well as medical or natural remedies, it is possible to manage symptoms and even cure the condition. If you suspect you may have internal hemorrhoids, it is important to consult with a healthcare professional for an accurate diagnosis and the best treatment plan for you.

Chapter Seven

External hemorrhoids

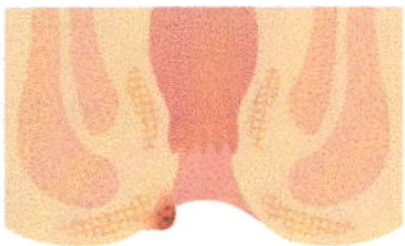

External hemorrhoids are a common condition that affects many people at some point in their lives. They are a type of varicose vein that develops in the anus and rectum.

Hemorrhoids are caused by increased pressure in the veins of the anus and rectum. This pressure can come from a variety of sources, including constipation, diarrhea, and pregnancy. When the pressure becomes too great, the veins in these areas can become swollen and bulge out, creating a hemorrhoid.

Symptoms of external hemorrhoids include itching, burning, and pain around the anus. They may also cause bleeding during bowel movements. In some cases, external hemorrhoids can become thrombosed, meaning they have formed a blood clot. This can cause severe pain and swelling.

Treatment for external hemorrhoids typically begins with lifestyle changes and over-the-counter medications. Eating a high-fiber diet, drinking plenty of water, and getting regular exercise can help to prevent constipation and reduce the pressure on the veins in the anus and rectum. Over-the-counter creams and ointments can also be used to alleviate itching and burning.

If these measures are not enough to control symptoms, a doctor may recommend more aggressive treatment options. One common treatment is rubber band ligation, which involves placing a small rubber band around the base of the hemorrhoid to cut off its blood supply. This causes the hemorrhoid to shrink and eventually fall off.

Another option is sclerotherapy, which involves injecting a solution into the hemorrhoid to shrink it. Surgical procedures, such as hemorrhoidectomy, may be necessary in severe cases.

In some cases, external hemorrhoids can be prevented by taking steps to reduce the pressure on the veins in the anus and rectum. This may include avoiding prolonged sitting or standing, losing weight if you are overweight, and avoiding straining during bowel movements.

While external hemorrhoids can be uncomfortable and even painful, they are typically not serious and can be treated effectively with lifestyle changes and over-the-counter medications. If your symptoms persist or worsen, it's important to see a doctor for proper diagnosis and treatment.

It's also important to note that hemorrhoids are a common condition and should not be ignored, if you suspect you have hemorrhoids, it's best to consult a doctor to find out the best treatment options for you.

In summary, External hemorrhoids are a common condition that affects many people, it's caused by increased pressure in the veins of the anus and rectum. Symptoms include itching, burning, and pain around the anus and in some cases bleeding during bowel movements. Treatment options include lifestyle changes, over-the-counter medications, rubber band ligation, sclerotherapy, and surgical procedures. Consult a doctor if you suspect you have hemorrhoids to find out the best treatment options for you.

Prolapsed Hemorrhoids

Hemorrhoids are a common medical condition that affects millions of people worldwide. They are caused by increased pressure on the veins in the anus or rectum, and can be caused by a variety of factors, including constipation, diarrhea, pregnancy, prolonged sitting, obesity, and genetics. Prolapsed hemorrhoids occur when internal hemorrhoids become swollen and protrude outside of the anus.Below we will explore the causes, symptoms, and treatment options for prolapsed hemorrhoids.

Causes of Prolapsed Hemorrhoids:

Prolapsed hemorrhoids are caused by increased pressure on the veins in the anus or rectum. This can be caused by a variety of factors, including constipation, diarrhea, pregnancy, prolonged sitting, obesity, and genetics. When the pressure becomes too great, internal hemorrhoids can become swollen and protrude outside of the anus, resulting in prolapsed hemorrhoids.

Symptoms of Prolapsed Hemorrhoids:

The most common symptom of prolapsed hemorrhoids is a lump or bulge outside of the anus. This can be accompanied by pain, itching, and bleeding during bowel movements. In some cases, the prolapsed hemorrhoid may need to be manually pushed back inside the anus, which can be uncomfortable or painful.

Treatment for Prolapsed Hemorrhoids:

Treatment for prolapsed hemorrhoids typically involves lifestyle changes, such as increasing fiber intake and exercising regularly to prevent constipation, as well as over-the-counter medications to relieve pain and itching. In some cases, prescription medications or surgery may be necessary to treat more severe cases of prolapsed hemorrhoids.

Self-Care:

Self-care measures can be effective in treating mild to moderate cases of prolapsed hemorrhoids. This may include taking warm baths or using a sitz bath to soothe the area, using over-the-counter creams or ointments to relieve pain and itching, and increasing fiber intake to prevent constipation.

Minimally Invasive Procedures:

Minimally invasive procedures, such as rubber band ligation or sclerotherapy, may be recommended for more severe cases of prolapsed hemorrhoids. These procedures involve the use of small bands or injections to cut off the blood supply to the hemorrhoid, causing it to shrink and fall off.

Surgery:

Surgery may be recommended in rare cases of severe or persistent prolapsed hemorrhoids. This may include hemorrhoidectomy, which involves the removal of the hemorrhoid, or stapled hemorrhoidopexy, which involves the use of a stapling device to reposition the hemorrhoid back inside the anus.

Thrombosed Hemorrhoids

Thrombosed hemorrhoids occur when a blood clot forms in a swollen vein in the anus or rectum.Below we will explore the causes, symptoms, and treatment options for thrombosed hemorrhoids.

Causes of Thrombosed Hemorrhoids:

Thrombosed hemorrhoids are caused by increased pressure on the veins in the anus or rectum. This can be caused by a variety of factors, including constipation, diarrhea, pregnancy, prolonged sitting, obesity, and genetics. When the pressure becomes too great, the veins can become swollen and a blood clot may form, resulting in thrombosed hemorrhoids.

Symptoms of Thrombosed Hemorrhoids:

The most common symptom of thrombosed hemorrhoids is a painful lump or swelling around the anus. This can be accompanied by itching, bleeding, and discomfort during bowel movements. In some cases, the thrombosed hemorrhoid may need to be manually removed, which can be very painful.

Treatment for Thrombosed Hemorrhoids:

Treatment for thrombosed hemorrhoids typically involves lifestyle changes, such as increasing fiber intake and exercising regularly to prevent constipation, as well as over-the-counter medications to relieve pain and itching. In some cases, prescription medications or surgery may be necessary to treat more severe cases of thrombosed hemorrhoids.

Self-Care:

Self-care measures can be effective in treating mild to moderate cases of thrombosed hemorrhoids. This may include taking warm baths or using a sitz bath to soothe the area, using over-the-counter creams or ointments to relieve pain and itching, and increasing fiber intake to prevent constipation.

Minimally Invasive Procedures:

Minimally invasive procedures, such as rubber band ligation or sclerotherapy, may be recommended for more severe cases of thrombosed hemorrhoids. These procedures involve the use of small bands or injections to cut off the blood supply to the hemorrhoid, causing it to shrink and fall off.

Surgery:

Surgery may be recommended in rare cases of severe or persistent thrombosed hemorrhoids. This may include hemorrhoidectomy, which involves the removal of the hemorrhoid, or stapled hemorrhoidopexy, which involves the use of a stapling device to reposition the hemorrhoid back inside the anus.

Chapter Eight

How can hemorrhoids be prevented?

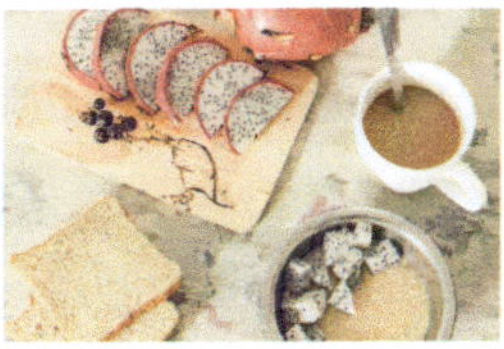

Hemorrhoids are a common condition that affects many people at some point in their lives. They are caused by the inflammation of the veins in the rectum and anus, and can be extremely uncomfortable and painful. However, the good news is that there are several things you can do to prevent hemorrhoids from developing in the first place.

One of the most important things you can do to prevent hemorrhoids is to maintain a healthy diet. Eating a diet that is high in fiber is essential for preventing constipation, which is one of the main causes of hemorrhoids. Fiber helps to keep the stools soft and bulky, making them easier to pass. Good sources of fiber include fruits, vegetables, whole grains, and legumes.

Another way to prevent hemorrhoids is to stay hydrated. Drinking plenty of water and other fluids can help to keep the stools soft and prevent constipation. It is recommended to drink at least eight glasses of water a day, but you may need more if you're active or live in a hot climate.

Exercise is also an important part of preventing hemorrhoids. Regular physical activity can help to promote regular bowel movements and can also help to improve circulation in the rectal area. Aim for at least 30 minutes of moderate exercise, such as brisk walking, jogging, cycling, or swimming, most days of the week.

Prolonged sitting or standing can also contribute to the development of hemorrhoids. It is important to take regular breaks throughout the day, and to get up and move around. Sitting for long periods of time can put pressure on the rectal veins and can cause them to become inflamed.

You can also prevent hemorrhoids by practicing good hygiene. Cleaning the rectal area gently after each bowel movement can help to prevent irritation and inflammation. It is also important to avoid using harsh soaps or toilet paper, as they can further irritate the rectal area.

If you are already experiencing hemorrhoids symptoms, it is important to avoid activities that can worsen them. Heavy lifting and strenuous exercise can put extra pressure on the rectal veins and can make hemorrhoids worse.

Finally, if you are pregnant, you are at a higher risk for developing hemorrhoids. This is due to the increased pressure on the rectal veins from the growing uterus. To prevent hemorrhoids during pregnancy, it is important to maintain a healthy diet, stay hydrated, and get regular exercise. You should also avoid prolonged sitting or standing, and practice good hygiene.

In summary, hemorrhoids can be prevented by maintaining a healthy diet high in fiber, staying hydrated, regular exercise, avoiding prolonged sitting or standing, practicing good hygiene, and avoiding activities that can worsen the symptoms if you already experiencing them. Pregnant women should also take extra care to prevent hemorrhoids during their pregnancy. Remember that it's always better to prevent hemorrhoids than to treat them, so take steps to maintain a healthy lifestyle and take care of your rectal and anal area.

Chapter Nine

How are hemorrhoids diagnosed?

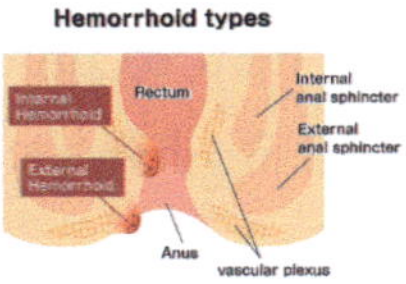

Hemorrhoids, also known as piles, are swollen veins in the lower rectum and anus. They can be a painful and uncomfortable condition, but the good news is that they are typically easy to diagnose. In this chapter, we'll go over the various methods that doctors use to diagnose hemorrhoids, so you can have a better understanding of what to expect if you ever need to see a doctor for this condition.

The first step in diagnosing hemorrhoids is usually a physical examination. The doctor will look at the anus and rectum to see if there are any visible signs of hemorrhoids, such as swelling or lumps. They may also use a tool called an anoscope, which is a short, hollow tube with a light on the end, to look inside the anus and rectum. This can help the doctor get a better view of the hemorrhoids and see if they are internal or external.

Another common diagnostic method is a digital rectal exam (DRE). During this exam, the doctor will gently insert a gloved finger into the rectum to feel for any lumps or other abnormalities. This can help the doctor determine the size and location of the hemorrhoids.

If the doctor suspects that the patient may have more serious problems, such as colon cancer, they may also recommend a colonoscopy. During this procedure, a thin, flexible tube with a camera on the end is inserted into the rectum and moved through the entire colon. This allows the doctor to get a detailed look at the entire colon, including any hemorrhoids, and can help rule out other conditions that may be causing similar symptoms.

Another test that can be used to diagnose hemorrhoids is a sigmoidoscopy. Similar to a colonoscopy, a sigmoidoscopy uses a thin tube with a camera on the end to examine the lower portion of the colon and rectum. This procedure can be used to find out if the hemorrhoids are causing any blockages or bleeding.

There are also several non-invasive tests that can be used to diagnose hemorrhoids. One of these is a stool test, which can detect blood in the stool. This can be a sign of hemorrhoids, as well as other conditions such as colon cancer. Another non-invasive test is a proctoscopy, which uses a short, lighted tube to examine the rectum and anus. This test can help the doctor detect any abnormal growths or swelling.

In some cases, a doctor may also recommend a Doppler-guided hemorrhoid artery ligation. This procedure uses a special tool to identify the blood vessels that are supplying blood to the hemorrhoids and then ties them off to reduce the blood flow to the hemorrhoids. This can help shrink the hemorrhoids and reduce symptoms such as pain and bleeding.

Overall, diagnosing hemorrhoids is typically a straightforward process. A physical examination, digital rectal exam, and possibly a colonoscopy or sigmoidoscopy are the most common methods used to diagnose hemorrhoids. Non-invasive tests such as stool tests and proctoscopy can also be used to help confirm the diagnosis. If you have any symptoms of hemorrhoids, such as itching, pain, or bleeding, it's important to see a doctor to have them properly diagnosed and treated.

In conclusion, Hemorrhoids are a common condition that can be diagnosed by a variety of methods. A physical examination and a digital rectal exam are the first step to diagnosis. If the doctor suspects more serious problems, such as colon cancer, they may recommend a colonoscopy or sigmoidoscopy.

Common Signs Of Hemorrhoids

Hemorrhoids are a common medical condition that affects millions of people worldwide. They are caused by increased pressure on the veins in the anus or rectum, and can be caused by a variety of factors, including constipation, diarrhea, pregnancy, prolonged sitting, obesity, and genet ics.Below we will explore the common signs of hemorrhoids, including symptoms and physical signs.

1. Pain or discomfort: One of the most common signs of hemorrhoids is pain or discomfort in the anal or rectal area. This can be caused by the swelling and inflammation of the veins in the area.

2. Itching: Itching in the anal or rectal area can also be a sign of hemorrhoids. This can be caused by the irritation of the skin around the anus due to the swelling and inflammation of the veins.

3. Bleeding: Hemorrhoids can also cause bleeding during bowel movements. This can be caused by the strain of passing stool, which can rupture the swollen veins in the anus or rectum.

4. Swelling: Swelling in the anal or rectal area is another common sign of hemorrhoids. This can be caused by the inflammation of the veins and the surrounding tissue.

5. Discomfort during bowel movements: Hemorrhoids can also cause discomfort or pain during bowel movements. This can be caused by the pressure on the veins in the anus or rectum when passing stool.

6. Lumps or bumps: In some cases, hemorrhoids can cause lumps or bumps to form around the anus or rectum. These can be painful and tender to the touch.

7. Leakage of feces: Hemorrhoids can also cause leakage of feces from the anus. This can be caused by the swelling and inflammation of the veins in the area, which can weaken the muscles that control bowel movements.

It is important to note that not all cases of hemorrhoids will have all of these symptoms. Some people may experience only a few of these symptoms, while others may not experience any symptoms at all. Additionally, other medical conditions can cause similar symptoms, so it is important to consult with a healthcare provider for an accurate diagnosis.

Treatment for hemorrhoids typically involves lifestyle changes, such as increasing fiber intake and exercising regularly to prevent constipation, as well as over-the-counter medications to relieve pain and itching. In some cases, prescription medications or surgery may be necessary to treat more severe cases of hemorrhoids.

Chapter Ten

How do you treat hemorrhoids?

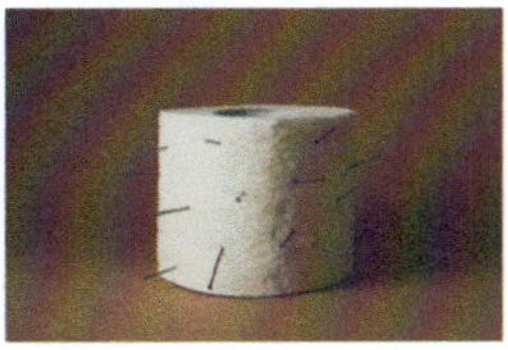

Hemorrhoids, also known as piles, are swollen veins in the lower rectum and anus. They can be caused by a variety of factors such as constipation, diarrhea, pregnancy, and a sedentary lifestyle. Hemorrhoids can be treated in a variety of ways, depending on the severity of the condition.

The first step in treating hemorrhoids is to address the underlying cause. For example, if constipation is the cause, then increasing your fiber intake and drinking plenty of water can help to soften stools and make them easier to pass. This can help to reduce the pressure on the hemorrhoids and prevent them from becoming worse.

Over-the-counter creams and ointments can also be used to relieve the symptoms of hemorrhoids. These products usually contain ingredients such as witch hazel, hydrocortisone, or lidocaine, which can help to soothe the itching and pain associated with hemorrhoids. They can also help to shrink the swollen veins and reduce inflammation.

For more severe cases of hemorrhoids, your doctor may recommend a procedure called rubber band ligation. During this procedure, a small rubber band is placed around the base of the hemorrhoid, cutting off the blood supply. This causes the hemorrhoid to shrink and eventually fall off. This procedure is typically done in the doctor's office and is relatively painless.

Another procedure that is used to treat hemorrhoids is called sclerotherapy. During this procedure, a chemical solution is injected into the hemorrhoid, causing it to shrink. This procedure is typically used for smaller hemorrhoids and is also relatively painless.

In some cases, surgery may be necessary to treat hemorrhoids. The most common surgical procedure is called a hemorrhoidectomy. During this procedure, the hemorrhoids are removed surgically. This procedure is typically used for larger and more severe hemorrhoids, and it is usually done under general anesthesia.

In addition to the above-mentioned treatment, some lifestyle changes that can help prevent hemorrhoids from developing or becoming worse include exercising regularly, maintaining a healthy diet, and avoiding prolonged sitting or standing.

Hemorrhoids can be treated in a variety of ways, and the treatment will depend on the severity of the condition. For mild cases, over-the-counter creams and ointments can provide relief from the symptoms. For more severe cases, rubber band ligation, sclerotherapy, or surgery may be necessary.

It's important to remember that hemorrhoids are a common condition and are not a serious health concern. However, if you are experiencing symptoms such as bleeding, severe pain, or a change in bowel habits, it is important to see a doctor for an examination. With proper treatment and lifestyle changes, hemorrhoids can be effectively managed.

The Importance Of Seeking Medical Advice If You Have Hemorrhoids

Hemorrhoids are a common medical condition that affects millions of people worldwide. They are caused by increased pressure on the veins in the anus or rectum, and can be caused by a variety of factors, including constipation, diarrhea, pregnancy, prolonged sitting, obesity, and genetics. While hemorrhoids can be uncomfortable and even painful, they are typically not a serious medical condition. However, it is important to seek medical advice if you have hemorrhoids.Below we will explore the importance of seeking medical advice if you have hemorrhoids.

1. Accurate diagnosis: There are several medical conditions that can cause symptoms similar to hemorrhoids, including anal fissures, rectal prolapse, and colorectal cancer. Seeking medical advice can help ensure an accurate diagnosis and appropriate treatment plan.

2. Effective treatment: While hemorrhoids can be managed with over-the-counter medications and lifestyle changes, more severe cases may require prescription medications or even surgery. A healthcare provider can provide guidance on the most effective treatment options for your specific case.

3. Management of symptoms: Hemorrhoids can be uncomfortable and even painful, and seeking medical advice can help manage symptoms. A healthcare provider can provide advice on how to relieve pain and itching and manage other symptoms.

4. Prevention of complications: In rare cases, complications can occur with hemorrhoids, including blood clots, thrombosis, and anemia. Seeking medical advice can help prevent these complications and ensure early treatment if they do occur.

5. Monitoring for changes: Hemorrhoids can sometimes lead to more serious medical conditions, such as colorectal cancer. A healthcare provider

can monitor for any changes or progression of symptoms, and provide appropriate medical care if needed.

Diagnostic Methods And Procedures Of Hemorrhoids

Hemorrhoids are a common medical condition that affects millions of people worldwide. They are caused by increased pressure on the veins in the anus or rectum, and can be caused by a variety of factors, including constipation, diarrhea, pregnancy, prolonged sitting, obesity, and genetics. While hemorrhoids can be uncomfortable and even painful, they are typically not a serious medical condition. However, in order to receive an accurate diagnosis and appropriate treatment plan, diagnostic methods and procedures may be necessary.Below we will explore the diagnostic methods and procedures of hemorrhoids.

1. Physical examination: A physical examination is usually the first step in diagnosing hemorrhoids. A healthcare provider will examine the anus and rectum for signs of hemorrhoids, such as swelling, inflammation, or lumps.

2. Digital rectal exam: A digital rectal exam may also be performed to check for hemorrhoids. During this exam, a healthcare provider will insert a lubricated, gloved finger into the anus to check for swelling or tenderness.

3. Anoscopy: An anoscopy is a procedure that allows a healthcare provider to view the inside of the anus and rectum using a small, lighted tube called an anoscope. This can help to identify the location and severity of hemorrhoids.

4. Sigmoidoscopy: A sigmoidoscopy is a procedure that allows a healthcare provider to view the inside of the rectum and lower colon using a long,

flexible tube called a sigmoidoscope. This can help to identify any other medical conditions that may be causing symptoms similar to hemorrhoids.

5. Colonoscopy: A colonoscopy is a procedure that allows a healthcare provider to view the inside of the entire colon using a long, flexible tube called a colonoscope. This may be recommended if there are concerns about more serious medical conditions, such as colorectal cancer.

6. Stool sample testing: Stool sample testing may also be performed to check for any other medical conditions that may be causing symptoms similar to hemorrhoids, such as infection or inflammation.

Topical Medications To Treat Hemorrhoids

Hemorrhoids are a common medical condition that affects millions of people worldwide. They are caused by increased pressure on the veins in the anus or rectum, and can be caused by a variety of factors, including constipation, diarrhea, pregnancy, prolonged sitting, obesity, and genetics. Topical medications are one of the most commonly used treatments for hemorrhoids.Below we will explore the different types of topical medications used to treat hemorrhoids, their benefits, and potential side effects.

Corticosteroids:

Corticosteroids are anti-inflammatory medications that can be applied topically to reduce swelling and inflammation in the affected area. They are commonly used to treat hemorrhoids that are painful or itchy. However, they should only be used for short periods of time, as prolonged use can lead to skin thinning and other side effects.

Local Anesthetics:

Local anesthetics are medications that can be applied topically to provide pain relief. They work by numbing the affected area and can be helpful in relieving pain associated with hemorrhoids. However, they should only be used for short periods of time, as prolonged use can lead to skin irritation and other side effects.

Vasoconstrictors:

Vasoconstrictors are medications that can be applied topically to reduce swelling and inflammation in the affected area. They work by constricting blood vessels, which can help to reduce bleeding and pain associated with hemorrhoids. However, they should only be used for short periods of time, as prolonged use can lead to skin irritation and other side effects.

Astringents:

Astringents are medications that can be applied topically to help dry out the affected area and reduce swelling. They work by constricting blood vessels and can be helpful in reducing pain associated with hemorrhoids. However, they should only be used for short periods of time, as prolonged use can lead to skin irritation and other side effects.

Moisturizers:

Moisturizers are medications that can be applied topically to help soothe and moisturize the affected area. They work by providing a protective barrier and can be helpful in reducing itching and irritation associated with hemorrhoids.

Oral Medications To Treat Hemorrhoids

Hemorrhoids are a common medical condition that affects millions of people worldwide. They are caused by increased pressure on the veins in the anus or rectum, and can be caused by a variety of factors, including constipation, diarrhea, pregnancy, prolonged sitting, obesity, and genetics. While topical medications are often used to treat hemorrhoids, oral medications can also be effective in relieving symptoms.Below we will explore the different types of oral medications used to treat hemorrhoids, their benefits, and potential side effects.

Analgesics:

Analgesics are pain-relieving medications that can be taken orally to relieve pain associated with hemorrhoids. They work by blocking pain signals to the brain and can be helpful in reducing discomfort and pain associated with hemorrhoids. Common analgesics used to treat hemorrhoids include acetaminophen and ibuprofen.

Anti-inflammatory Medications:

Anti-inflammatory medications can be taken orally to reduce swelling and inflammation in the affected area. They work by blocking the production of inflammatory substances in the body and can be helpful in reducing pain and swelling associated with hemorrhoids. Common anti-inflammatory medications used to treat hemorrhoids include aspirin and non-steroidal anti-inflammatory drugs (NSAIDs) such as ibuprofen.

Stool Softeners:

Stool softeners are medications that can be taken orally to help soften the stool and make bowel movements easier. They work by increasing the amount of water in the stool, making it easier to pass. Stool softeners can be helpful in reducing the strain and pressure on the anus and rectum, which can help to reduce the risk of hemorrhoids. Common stool softeners used to treat hemorrhoids include docusate sodium.

Fiber Supplements:

Fiber supplements are medications that can be taken orally to increase the amount of fiber in the diet. They work by adding bulk to the stool, making it easier to pass. Fiber supplements can be helpful in reducing the risk of constipation and diarrhea, which can contribute to the development of hemorrhoids. Common fiber supplements used to treat hemorrhoids include psyllium husk and methylcellulose.

Venotonic Agents:

Venotonic agents are medications that can be taken orally to improve the tone and elasticity of the veins in the anus and rectum. They work by improving blood flow and reducing the pressure on the veins. Venotonic agents can be helpful in reducing the risk of hemorrhoids and improving symptoms associated with hemorrhoids. Common venotonic agents used to treat hemorrhoids include diosmin and hesperidin.

Sclerotherapy To Treat Hemorrhoids

Hemorrhoids are a common medical condition that affects millions of people worldwide. They are caused by increased pressure on the veins in the anus or rectum, and can be caused by a variety of factors, including constipation, diarrhea, pregnancy, prolonged sitting, obesity, and genetics. Sclerotherapy is a minimally invasive procedure used to treat hemorrhoid s.Below we will explore what sclerotherapy is, how it works, and its benefits and potential risks.

What is Sclerotherapy?

Sclerotherapy is a minimally invasive procedure that involves injecting a chemical solution into the hemorrhoid. The chemical solution causes the vein to collapse and eventually disappear, reducing the size of the hemorrhoid.

How does Sclerotherapy work?

During sclerotherapy, a healthcare provider will inject a chemical solution into the hemorrhoid. The chemical solution causes the vein to become irritated and eventually collapse, reducing the size of the hemorrhoid. Over time, the collapsed vein is absorbed by the body and disappears.

Benefits of Sclerotherapy:

Sclerotherapy is a minimally invasive procedure that can be performed in a healthcare provider's office or clinic. It is a quick and relatively painless procedure, with most patients experiencing only minor discomfort during the injection. Sclerotherapy is also an effective treatment option for hemorrhoids, with many patients experiencing significant reduction in hemorrhoid size and symptoms after the procedure.

Risks of Sclerotherapy:

While sclerotherapy is generally considered safe, there are some potential risks and side effects associated with the procedure. These may include bleeding, infection, and allergic reactions to the chemical solution. In some cases, the injection may be painful, and some patients may experience a burning or itching sensation after the procedure.

Who is a candidate for Sclerotherapy?

Sclerotherapy may be recommended for patients with internal hemorrhoids that are causing significant discomfort or bleeding. It is generally not recommended for patients with external hemorrhoids or those with severe hemorrhoids that require surgical intervention.

How is Sclerotherapy performed?

During sclerotherapy, the patient will lie on their side with their knees bent. The healthcare provider will then insert a small, thin needle into the hemorrhoid and inject the chemical solution. The procedure usually takes only a few minutes to complete, and patients can typically return to their normal activities immediately after the procedure.

Rubber Band Ligation To Treat Hemorrhoids

Hemorrhoids are a common medical condition that affects millions of people worldwide. They are caused by increased pressure on the veins in the anus or rectum, and can be caused by a variety of factors, including constipation, diarrhea, pregnancy, prolonged sitting, obesity, and genetics. Rubber band ligation is a minimally invasive procedure used to treat hemorrhoids.Below we will explore what rubber band ligation is, how it works, and its benefits and potential risks.

What is Rubber Band Ligation?

Rubber band ligation is a minimally invasive procedure that involves placing a rubber band around the base of the hemorrhoid. The rubber band cuts off the blood supply to the hemorrhoid, causing it to shrink and eventually fall off.

How does Rubber Band Ligation work?

During rubber band ligation, a healthcare provider will place a small, tight rubber band around the base of the hemorrhoid. The rubber band cuts off the blood supply to the hemorrhoid, causing it to shrink and eventually fall off. Over time, the remaining tissue is absorbed by the body and the hemorrhoid disappears.

Benefits of Rubber Band Ligation:

Rubber band ligation is a minimally invasive procedure that can be performed in a healthcare provider's office or clinic. It is a quick and relatively painless procedure, with most patients experiencing only minor discomfort during the placement of the rubber band. Rubber band ligation is also an effective treatment option for hemorrhoids, with many patients experiencing significant reduction in hemorrhoid size and symptoms after the procedure.

Risks of Rubber Band Ligation:

While rubber band ligation is generally considered safe, there are some potential risks and side effects associated with the procedure. These may include bleeding, infection, and pain or discomfort during bowel movements. In some cases, the rubber band may slip off the hemorrhoid and require additional treatment.

Who is a candidate for Rubber Band Ligation?

Rubber band ligation may be recommended for patients with internal hemorrhoids that are causing significant discomfort or bleeding. It is generally not recommended for patients with external hemorrhoids or those with severe hemorrhoids that require surgical intervention.

How is Rubber Band Ligation performed?

During rubber band ligation, the patient will lie on their side with their knees bent. The healthcare provider will then use an anoscope to visualize the hemorrhoid and place a small, tight rubber band around the base of the hemorrhoid. The procedure usually takes only a few minutes to complete, and patients can typically return to their normal activities immediately after the procedure.

Infrared Coagulatio To Treat Hemorrhoidsn

Hemorrhoids are a common medical condition that affects millions of people worldwide. They are caused by increased pressure on the veins in the anus or rectum, and can be caused by a variety of factors, including constipation, diarrhea, pregnancy, prolonged sitting, obesity, and genetics. Infrared coagulation (IRC) is a minimally invasive procedure used to treat hemorrhoids.Below we will explore what IRC is, how it works, and its benefits and potential risks.

What is Infrared Coagulation?

Infrared coagulation (IRC) is a minimally invasive procedure that uses infrared light to coagulate the blood vessels in the hemorrhoid. This causes the hemorrhoid to shrink and eventually disappear.

How does Infrared Coagulation work?

During IRC, a healthcare provider will use a small probe to deliver infrared light to the hemorrhoid. The infrared light coagulates the blood vessels in the hemorrhoid, causing it to shrink and eventually disappear. Over time, the remaining tissue is absorbed by the body and the hemorrhoid disappears.

Benefits of Infrared Coagulation:

IRC is a minimally invasive procedure that can be performed in a health-care provider's office or clinic. It is a quick and relatively painless procedure, with most patients experiencing only minor discomfort during the delivery of the infrared light. IRC is also an effective treatment option for hemorrhoids, with many patients experiencing significant reduction in hemorrhoid size and symptoms after the procedure.

Risks of Infrared Coagulation:

While IRC is generally considered safe, there are some potential risks and side effects associated with the procedure. These may include bleeding, infection, and pain or discomfort during bowel movements. In some cases, multiple treatments may be required to achieve the desired results.

Who is a candidate for Infrared Coagulation?

IRC may be recommended for patients with internal hemorrhoids that are causing significant discomfort or bleeding. It is generally not recommended for patients with external hemorrhoids or those with severe hemorrhoids that require surgical intervention.

How is Infrared Coagulation performed?

During IRC, the patient will lie on their side with their knees bent. The healthcare provider will then use a small probe to deliver infrared light to the hemorrhoid. The procedure usually takes only a few minutes to complete, and patients can typically return to their normal activities immediately after the procedure.

Surgical Treatment Options To Treat Hemorrhoids

Hemorrhoids are a common medical condition that affects millions of people worldwide. They are caused by increased pressure on the veins in the anus or rectum, and can be caused by a variety of factors, including constipation, diarrhea, pregnancy, prolonged sitting, obesity, and genetics. While non-surgical treatment options are often effective in treating hemorrhoids, surgical options may be necessary in some cases.Below we will explore the different surgical treatment options available to treat hemorrhoids, their benefits, and potential risks.

Hemorrhoidectomy:

Hemorrhoidectomy is a surgical procedure used to remove internal or external hemorrhoids. It is usually performed under general anesthesia and involves cutting away the hemorrhoid tissue. This procedure is typically reserved for patients with severe or persistent hemorrhoids that have not responded to other treatments.

Benefits of Hemorrhoidectomy:

Hemorrhoidectomy is a highly effective treatment option for severe or persistent hemorrhoids. It can provide long-term relief from symptoms and prevent the recurrence of hemorrhoids.

Risks of Hemorrhoidectomy:

While hemorrhoidectomy is generally considered safe, there are some potential risks and side effects associated with the procedure. These may include bleeding, infection, and pain or discomfort during bowel movements. Additionally, recovery from hemorrhoidectomy can be uncomfortable and may require several weeks of rest and recovery.

Stapled Hemorrhoidopexy:

Stapled hemorrhoidopexy, also known as stapling, is a surgical procedure that involves using a special stapling device to remove excess tissue and create a smaller, less painful hemorrhoid. This procedure is usually performed under general anesthesia and is typically reserved for patients with internal hemorrhoids.

Benefits of Stapled Hemorrhoidopexy:

Stapled hemorrhoidopexy is a less invasive procedure than hemorrhoidectomy and can provide long-term relief from symptoms. Recovery time is usually shorter than with hemorrhoidectomy, and there is less pain and discomfort during recovery.

Risks of Stapled Hemorrhoidopexy:

While stapled hemorrhoidopexy is generally considered safe, there are some potential risks and side effects associated with the procedure. These may include bleeding, infection, and pain or discomfort during bowel movements. Additionally, there is a risk of recurrence with stapled hemorrhoidopexy, as the procedure does not remove the hemorrhoid tissue.

Doppler Guided Hemorrhoidal Artery Ligation (DGHAL):

Doppler guided hemorrhoidal artery ligation (DGHAL) is a minimally invasive surgical procedure that involves using a special probe to identify and ligate the hemorrhoidal arteries. This procedure is typically performed under local anesthesia and is usually reserved for patients with internal hemorrhoids.

Benefits of DGHAL:

DGHAL is a minimally invasive procedure that can provide long-term relief from symptoms. It is associated with less pain and discomfort during recovery than hemorrhoidectomy and stapled hemorrhoidopexy.

Risks of DGHAL:

While DGHAL is generally considered safe, there are some potential risks and side effects associated with the procedure. These may include bleeding, infection, and pain or discomfort during bowel movements. Additionally, there is a risk of recurrence with DGHAL, as the procedure does not remove the hemorrhoid tissue.

Hemorrhoidectomy To Treat Hemorrhoids

Hemorrhoids are a common medical condition that affects millions of people worldwide. They are caused by increased pressure on the veins in the anus or rectum, and can be caused by a variety of factors, including constipation, diarrhea, pregnancy, prolonged sitting, obesity, and genetics. While non-surgical treatment options are often effective in treating hemorrhoids, surgical options may be necessary in some cases. Hemorrhoidectomy is one such surgical option, andBelow we will explore what hemorrhoidectomy is, how it works, and its benefits and potential risks.

What is Hemorrhoidectomy?

Hemorrhoidectomy is a surgical procedure used to remove internal or external hemorrhoids. It is usually performed under general anesthesia and involves cutting away the hemorrhoid tissue. This procedure is typically reserved for patients with severe or persistent hemorrhoids that have not responded to other treatments.

How does Hemorrhoidectomy work?

During hemorrhoidectomy, the patient will be placed under general anesthesia. The healthcare provider will then make incisions around the hemorrhoid and remove the excess tissue. The wound is then closed with sutures. The procedure usually takes between 30 minutes and an hour to complete.

Benefits of Hemorrhoidectomy:

Hemorrhoidectomy is a highly effective treatment option for severe or persistent hemorrhoids. It can provide long-term relief from symptoms and prevent the recurrence of hemorrhoids. Additionally, hemorrhoidectomy is associated with a low rate of recurrence, meaning that most patients will not need further treatment for their hemorrhoids.

Risks of Hemorrhoidectomy:

While hemorrhoidectomy is generally considered safe, there are some potential risks and side effects associated with the procedure. These may include bleeding, infection, and pain or discomfort during bowel movements. Additionally, recovery from hemorrhoidectomy can be uncomfortable and may require several weeks of rest and recovery. Some patients may also experience difficulty with bowel movements or incontinence after the procedure.

Who is a candidate for Hemorrhoidectomy?

Hemorrhoidectomy may be recommended for patients with severe or persistent hemorrhoids that have not responded to non-surgical treatment options. It is generally not recommended for patients with external hemorrhoids or those with less severe hemorrhoids that can be treated with non-surgical options.

How is Hemorrhoidectomy performed?

During hemorrhoidectomy, the patient will be placed under general anesthesia. The healthcare provider will then make incisions around the hemorrhoid and remove the excess tissue. The wound is then closed with sutures. The procedure usually takes between 30 minutes and an hour to complete. Patients will typically be discharged from the hospital on the same day as the procedure.

Stapled Hemorrhoidopexy To Treat Hemorrhoids

Hemorrhoids are a common medical condition that affects millions of people worldwide. They are caused by increased pressure on the veins in the anus or rectum and can be caused by a variety of factors, including constipation, diarrhea, pregnancy, prolonged sitting, obesity, and genetics. While non-surgical treatment options are often effective in treating hemorrhoids, surgical options may be necessary in some cases. Stapled hemorrhoidopexy is one such surgical option, andBelow we will explore what stapled hemorrhoidopexy is, how it works, and its benefits and potential risks.

What is Stapled Hemorrhoidopexy?

Stapled hemorrhoidopexy, also known as stapling, is a surgical procedure that involves using a special stapling device to remove excess tissue and create a smaller, less painful hemorrhoid. This procedure is usually performed under general anesthesia and is typically reserved for patients with internal hemorrhoids.

How does Stapled Hemorrhoidopexy work?

During stapled hemorrhoidopexy, the patient will be placed under general anesthesia. The healthcare provider will then use a stapling device to remove excess tissue and create a smaller, less painful hemorrhoid. This procedure is less invasive than traditional hemorrhoidectomy and is associated with less pain and discomfort during recovery.

Benefits of Stapled Hemorrhoidopexy:

Stapled hemorrhoidopexy is a less invasive procedure than hemorrhoidectomy and can provide long-term relief from symptoms. Recovery time is usually shorter than with hemorrhoidectomy, and there is less pain and discomfort during recovery. Additionally, stapled hemorrhoidopexy is associated with a low rate of recurrence, meaning that most patients will not need further treatment for their hemorrhoids.

Risks of Stapled Hemorrhoidopexy:

While stapled hemorrhoidopexy is generally considered safe, there are some potential risks and side effects associated with the procedure. These may include bleeding, infection, and pain or discomfort during bowel movements. Additionally, there is a risk of recurrence with stapled hemorrhoidopexy, as the procedure does not remove the hemorrhoid tissue.

Who is a candidate for Stapled Hemorrhoidopexy?

Stapled hemorrhoidopexy may be recommended for patients with internal hemorrhoids that are causing significant discomfort or bleeding. It is generally not recommended for patients with external hemorrhoids or those with severe hemorrhoids that require surgical intervention.

How is Stapled Hemorrhoidopexy performed?

During stapled hemorrhoidopexy, the patient will be placed under general anesthesia. The healthcare provider will then use a stapling device to remove excess tissue and create a smaller, less painful hemorrhoid. The procedure usually takes between 30 minutes and an hour to complete. Patients will typically be discharged from the hospital on the same day as the procedure.

Laser Hemorrhoid Surgery To Treat Hemorrhoids

Hemorrhoids are a common medical condition that affects millions of people worldwide. They are caused by increased pressure on the veins in the anus or rectum and can be caused by a variety of factors, including constipation, diarrhea, pregnancy, prolonged sitting, obesity, and genetics. While non-surgical treatment options are often effective in treating hemorrhoids, surgical options may be necessary in some cases. Laser hemorrhoid surgery is one such surgical option, andBelow we will explore what laser hemorrhoid surgery is, how it works, and its benefits and potential risks.

What is Laser Hemorrhoid Surgery?

Laser hemorrhoid surgery is a surgical procedure used to remove internal or external hemorrhoids. It is a minimally invasive procedure that uses a laser to remove the hemorrhoid tissue. This procedure is usually performed under general anesthesia and is typically reserved for patients with internal hemorrhoids.

How does Laser Hemorrhoid Surgery work?

During laser hemorrhoid surgery, the patient will be placed under general anesthesia. The healthcare provider will then use a laser to remove the hemorrhoid tissue. This procedure is less invasive than traditional hemorrhoidectomy and is associated with less pain and discomfort during recovery.

Benefits of Laser Hemorrhoid Surgery:

Laser hemorrhoid surgery is a minimally invasive procedure that can provide long-term relief from hemorrhoid symptoms. It is associated with less pain and discomfort during recovery than hemorrhoidectomy and stapled hemorrhoidopexy. Additionally, laser hemorrhoid surgery is associated with a low rate of recurrence, meaning that most patients will not need further treatment for their hemorrhoids.

Risks of Laser Hemorrhoid Surgery:

While laser hemorrhoid surgery is generally considered safe, there are some potential risks and side effects associated with the procedure. These may include bleeding, infection, and pain or discomfort during bowel movements. Additionally, there is a risk of recurrence with laser hemorrhoid surgery, as the procedure does not remove the hemorrhoid tissue.

Who is a candidate for Laser Hemorrhoid Surgery?

Laser hemorrhoid surgery may be recommended for patients with internal hemorrhoids that are causing significant discomfort or bleeding. It is generally not recommended for patients with external hemorrhoids or those with severe hemorrhoids that require surgical intervention.

How is Laser Hemorrhoid Surgery performed?

During laser hemorrhoid surgery, the patient will be placed under general anesthesia. The healthcare provider will then use a laser to remove the hemorrhoid tissue. The procedure usually takes between 30 minutes and an hour to complete. Patients will typically be discharged from the hospital on the same day as the procedure.

When To Consider Surgery To Treat Hemorrhoids

Hemorrhoids are a common medical condition that affects millions of people worldwide. They are caused by increased pressure on the veins in the anus or rectum and can be caused by a variety of factors, including constipation, diarrhea, pregnancy, prolonged sitting, obesity, and genetics. While non-surgical treatment options are often effective in treating hemorrhoids, surgical options may be necessary in some cases.Below we will explore when to consider surgery to treat hemorrhoids.

When to Consider Surgery:

Surgery for hemorrhoids may be recommended if other treatments have failed or if the hemorrhoids are causing significant discomfort or bleeding. The decision to undergo surgery will depend on the severity of the hemorrhoids, the patient's medical history, and their individual needs and preferences.

Surgical Options:

There are several surgical options for treating hemorrhoids, including traditional hemorrhoidectomy, stapled hemorrhoidopexy, laser hemorrhoid surgery, and others. The specific surgical option will depend on the individual patient's needs and the recommendations of their healthcare provider.

Traditional Hemorrhoidectomy:

Traditional hemorrhoidectomy is a surgical procedure that involves removing the hemorrhoid tissue. It is typically reserved for patients with severe or persistent hemorrhoids that have not responded to other treatments. Recovery from traditional hemorrhoidectomy can be uncomfortable and may require several weeks of rest and recovery.

Stapled Hemorrhoidopexy:

Stapled hemorrhoidopexy is a minimally invasive surgical procedure that uses a special stapling device to remove excess tissue and create a smaller, less painful hemorrhoid. Recovery time is usually shorter than with traditional hemorrhoidectomy, and there is less pain and discomfort during recovery.

Laser Hemorrhoid Surgery:

Laser hemorrhoid surgery is a minimally invasive surgical procedure that uses a laser to remove the hemorrhoid tissue. It is associated with less pain and discomfort during recovery than traditional hemorrhoidectomy and stapled hemorrhoidopexy. However, it is generally not recommended for patients with severe hemorrhoids or those with external hemorrhoids.

Other Surgical Options:

There are several other surgical options for treating hemorrhoids, including sclerotherapy, rubber band ligation, and infrared coagulation. These procedures are typically less invasive than traditional hemorrhoidectomy and may be recommended for patients with less severe hemorrhoids.

Risks of Surgery:

While surgical options for treating hemorrhoids are generally considered safe, there are some potential risks and side effects associated with the procedures. These may include bleeding, infection, and pain or discomfort during recovery. Additionally, there is a risk of recurrence with some surgical options, meaning that the hemorrhoids may return after the procedure.

Chapter Eleven

Alternative treatments for hemorrhoids

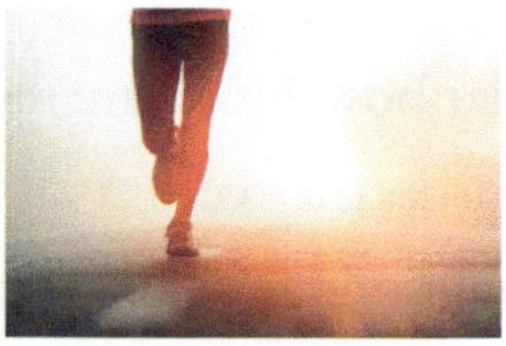

Hemorrhoids, also known as piles, are swollen veins in the lower rectum and anus. They can be caused by a variety of factors, including straining during bowel movements, obesity, and pregnancy. Hemorrhoids can be quite uncomfortable, causing symptoms such as itching, burning, and pain.

While there are several medical treatments for hemorrhoids, such as over-the-counter creams and surgery, many people prefer to try alternative treatments first. Here are a few alternative treatment options for hemorrhoids:

Topical herbal treatments: There are several herbs that have been traditionally used to treat hemorrhoids. Witch hazel, for example, has astringent properties that can help to shrink swollen blood vessels. Other herbs that may be helpful include aloe vera, horse chestnut, and calendula. These herbs can be found in a variety of forms, such as creams, ointments, and suppositories.

Sitz baths: A sitz bath is a shallow bath that is specifically designed to soothe hemorrhoids. To do a sitz bath, simply fill a bathtub with a few inches of warm water and sit in it for 10-15 minutes. The warm water can help to reduce inflammation and discomfort. Some people like to add Epsom salts or baking soda to the water for added relief.

Fiber-rich diet: Eating a diet that is high in fiber can help to prevent constipation, which is one of the main causes of hemorrhoids. Fiber can be found in fruits, vegetables, whole grains, and legumes. Additionally, drinking plenty of water can also help to prevent constipation.

Exercise: Regular exercise can help to promote regular bowel movements and can also help to reduce the pressure on the veins in the rectum and anus. Activities such as brisk walking, cycling, and swimming are all good options.

Avoid straining: Straining during bowel movements can put a lot of pressure on the veins in the rectum and anus, which can lead to hemorrhoids. To avoid straining, make sure to take your time when using the bathroom, and try to relax as much as possible.

Yoga and meditation: Yoga and meditation can be beneficial for reducing stress, which can contribute to the development of hemorrhoids. Certain yoga poses can also help to strengthen the muscles in the rectum and anus, which can help to prevent hemorrhoids from forming.

Acupuncture: Acupuncture is an ancient Chinese healing technique that involves the insertion of thin needles into the skin at specific points on the body. Some research suggests that acupuncture may be effective for treating hemorrhoids, although more research is needed to confirm these findings.

It's important to note that alternative treatments may not be effective for everyone, and if your symptoms persist or worsen, you should consult with a healthcare professional. Also, before trying any alternative treatment, it's important to consult with a healthcare professional to make sure it's safe for you.

In conclusion, hemorrhoids can be a painful and uncomfortable condition, but there are several alternative treatment options available. From topical herbal treatments, to sitz baths, to dietary changes, there are many ways to alleviate the symptoms of hemorrhoids. While these treatments may not work for everyone, they can be a good starting point for those who prefer to try more natural remedies before turning to more invasive options.

Preventing Hemorrhoids

While there are effective treatments for hemorrhoids, prevention is always the best course of action.Below we will explore some ways to prevent hemorrhoids from occurring in the first place.

Diet:

Diet plays a crucial role in preventing hemorrhoids. Eating a diet rich in fiber can help prevent constipation, which is a major risk factor for hemorrhoids. Foods such as fruits, vegetables, and whole grains are all good sources of fiber. Additionally, it is important to stay hydrated and drink plenty of water to help keep bowel movements soft and regular.

Exercise:

Regular exercise is another important way to prevent hemorrhoids. Exercise can help improve bowel function and reduce the risk of constipation. Additionally, regular exercise can help promote overall health and reduce the risk of obesity, which is another risk factor for hemorrhoids.

Avoid Prolonged Sitting:

Prolonged sitting can increase the pressure on the veins in the rectal area and increase the risk of hemorrhoids. It is important to take frequent breaks when sitting for long periods of time, and to try to incorporate movement into your daily routine. For example, taking short walks during your lunch break or standing up and stretching periodically throughout the day.

Good Bathroom Habits:

Good bathroom habits can also help prevent hemorrhoids. It is important to avoid straining during bowel movements, which can increase the pressure on the veins in the rectal area. One way to avoid straining is to avoid sitting on the toilet for long periods of time. It is also important to respond to the urge to have a bowel movement as soon as possible, as delaying can lead to constipation and increased pressure on the veins.

Maintain a Healthy Weight:

Maintaining a healthy weight is important for preventing hemorrhoids. Obesity is a major risk factor for hemorrhoids, as it increases the pressure on the veins in the rectal area. Eating a healthy diet and getting regular exercise can help maintain a healthy weight and reduce the risk of hemorrhoids.

Avoiding Straining:

Straining during bowel movements is a major risk factor for hemorrhoids. To avoid straining, it is important to respond to the urge to have a bowel movement as soon as possible. Additionally, it may be helpful to elevate your feet while on the toilet, which can help reduce the need to strain.

Dietary Changes And Fiber Intake

Dietary changes and increasing fiber intake are important factors in preventing and managing a variety of health conditions, including hemorrhoids. Hemorrhoids are a common medical condition that affects millions of people worldwide. They are caused by increased pressure on the veins in the anus or rectum and can be caused by a variety of factors, including constipation, diarrhea, pregnancy, prolonged sitting, obesity, and genetics.Below we will explore the role of dietary changes and fiber intake in preventing and managing hemorrhoids.

The Role of Fiber:

Fiber is an important nutrient that plays a crucial role in maintaining bowel health. Fiber is a type of carbohydrate that is not digested by the body, but instead passes through the digestive system largely intact. This can help keep the bowel movements soft and regular, reducing the risk of constipation and hemorrhoids.

There are two types of fiber: soluble and insoluble. Soluble fiber dissolves in water and forms a gel-like substance in the digestive system, while insoluble fiber does not dissolve in water and helps to add bulk to the stool. Both types of fiber are important for maintaining bowel health and preventing hemorrhoids.

Sources of Fiber:

Fiber can be found in a variety of foods, including fruits, vegetables, whole grains, and legumes. Some examples of high-fiber foods include:

- Apples
- Berries
- Oranges

- Carrots
- Broccoli
- Spinach
- Whole grain breads and cereals
- Brown rice
- Lentils
- Beans

Increasing Fiber Intake:

Increasing fiber intake is an important part of preventing and managing hemorrhoids. The American Heart Association recommends that adults consume at least 25 grams of fiber per day for women and 38 grams per day for men. However, many people do not consume enough fiber in their diets.

There are several ways to increase fiber intake. One way is to incorporate more fruits and vegetables into the diet. For example, adding a serving of fruit to breakfast and snacks, and adding vegetables to meals can help increase fiber intake. Choosing whole grain breads and cereals, brown rice, and quinoa instead of refined grains can also help increase fiber intake. Additionally, incorporating legumes such as beans and lentils into meals can provide an additional source of fiber.

Potential Benefits of Fiber:

Increasing fiber intake can have several potential benefits, including:

- 2. Preventing constipation: Constipation is a major risk factor for hemorrhoids, and increasing fiber intake can help keep bowel movements soft and regular, reducing the risk of constipation.

- 3. Promoting weight loss: High-fiber foods can help keep you feeling full, reducing the risk of overeating and promoting weight loss.

- 4. Lowering cholesterol: Soluble fiber can help lower cholesterol levels, reducing the risk of heart disease.

- 5. Reducing the risk of diabetes: High-fiber diets have been shown to reduce the risk of developing type 2 diabetes.

Regular Exercise

Regular exercise is an important factor in maintaining overall health and preventing a variety of health conditions, including hemorrhoids. Below we will explore the role of regular exercise in preventing and managing hemorrhoids.

The Role of Exercise:

Exercise plays a crucial role in maintaining overall health and preventing a variety of health conditions, including hemorrhoids. Exercise can help improve bowel function and reduce the risk of constipation, which is a major risk factor for hemorrhoids. Additionally, regular exercise can help promote overall health and reduce the risk of obesity, which is another risk factor for hemorrhoids.

Types of Exercise:

There are several types of exercise that can be beneficial for preventing and managing hemorrhoids, including:

- Aerobic exercise: Aerobic exercise, such as walking, jogging, swimming, or cycling, can help improve overall cardiovascular health and promote weight loss, both of which can reduce the risk of hemorrhoids.

- Resistance training: Resistance training, such as weight lifting or bodyweight exercises, can help strengthen the muscles in the pelvic area, reducing the risk of hemorrhoids.

- Yoga or Pilates: Yoga or Pilates can help improve flexibility and strengthen the muscles in the pelvic area, reducing the risk of hemorrhoids.

Benefits of Exercise:

Regular exercise can have several potential benefits, including:

- Improving bowel function: Exercise can help improve bowel function, reducing the risk of constipation and hemorrhoids.

- Promoting weight loss: Regular exercise can help promote weight loss, reducing the risk of obesity and the associated risk of hemorrhoids.

- Improving cardiovascular health: Regular exercise can help improve overall cardiovascular health, reducing the risk of heart disease and other health conditions.

- Reducing stress: Regular exercise can help reduce stress and improve mental health.

Incorporating Exercise into Daily Routine:

Incorporating exercise into daily routine can be challenging, but there are several ways to make it easier. One way is to find an exercise buddy or join a group fitness class, which can provide motivation and accountability. Additionally, it is important to choose activities that are enjoyable and sustainable, such as walking, cycling, or swimming. Finding time in the day to exercise, such as before or after work or during lunch breaks, can also help make regular exercise a part of daily routine.

Maintaining Healthy Bowel Habits

Maintaining healthy bowel habits is an important factor in preventing and managing a variety of health conditions, including hemorrhoids.

Below we will explore the importance of maintaining healthy bowel habits and how to do so.

The Importance of Healthy Bowel Habits:

Maintaining healthy bowel habits is important for a variety of reasons. It can help prevent constipation, which is a major risk factor for hemorrhoids. Additionally, healthy bowel habits can help reduce the risk of other health conditions, such as diverticulitis and colon cancer. Healthy bowel habits can also promote overall health and wellbeing.

Tips for Maintaining Healthy Bowel Habits:

There are several tips that can help maintain healthy bowel habits, including:

Responding to the urge to have a bowel movement:

Responding to the urge to have a bowel movement as soon as possible can help prevent constipation and reduce the risk of hemorrhoids. Delaying bowel movements can lead to constipation and increased pressure on the veins in the rectal area.

Avoiding straining:

Straining during bowel movements can increase the pressure on the veins in the rectal area and increase the risk of hemorrhoids. To avoid straining, it is important to respond to the urge to have a bowel movement as soon as possible. Additionally, it may be helpful to elevate your feet while on the toilet, which can help reduce the need to strain.

Drinking plenty of water:

Drinking plenty of water can help keep bowel movements soft and regular, reducing the risk of constipation and hemorrhoids.

Eating a high-fiber diet:

Eating a high-fiber diet can help keep bowel movements soft and regular, reducing the risk of constipation and hemorrhoids. Foods such as fruits, vegetables, whole grains, and legumes are all good sources of fiber.

Getting regular exercise:

Regular exercise can help improve bowel function and reduce the risk of constipation and hemorrhoids.

Maintaining a healthy weight:

Maintaining a healthy weight is important for preventing hemorrhoids, as obesity is a major risk factor for the condition.

Avoiding prolonged sitting:

Prolonged sitting can increase the pressure on the veins in the rectal area and increase the risk of hemorrhoids. It is important to take frequent breaks when sitting for long periods of time and to try to incorporate movement into your daily routine.

Avoiding excessive use of laxatives:

Excessive use of laxatives can lead to dependence and can actually worsen constipation over time. It is important to only use laxatives as directed by a healthcare provider.

Avoiding Prolonged Sitting

Avoiding prolonged sitting is an important factor in maintaining overall health and preventing a variety of health conditions, including hemorrhoids

Below we will explore the importance of avoiding prolonged sitting and how to do so.

The Role of Prolonged Sitting:

Prolonged sitting can increase the pressure on the veins in the rectal area and increase the risk of hemorrhoids. Additionally, prolonged sitting can lead to other health conditions, such as back pain and poor posture. Prolonged sitting is a common occurrence in today's society due to increased sedentary lifestyles and desk jobs.

Tips for Avoiding Prolonged Sitting:

There are several tips that can help avoid prolonged sitting, including:

Taking frequent breaks:

Taking frequent breaks when sitting for long periods of time can help reduce the pressure on the veins in the rectal area and reduce the risk of hemorrhoids. It is recommended to take a break at least once per hour and to incorporate movement into your daily routine.

Standing while working:

Standing while working can help reduce the risk of hemorrhoids and other health conditions associated with prolonged sitting. Many workplaces now offer standing desks or adjustable desks that can be used in either a sitting or standing position.

Walking during breaks:

Walking during breaks can help reduce the pressure on the veins in the rectal area and reduce the risk of hemorrhoids. It is recommended to take a short walk during breaks or lunchtime to incorporate movement into your daily routine.

Using a stability ball:

Using a stability ball instead of a traditional office chair can help improve posture and reduce the risk of hemorrhoids. Additionally, sitting on a stability ball can help engage the core muscles and improve overall health and wellbeing.

Incorporating movement into daily routine:

Incorporating movement into daily routine can help reduce the risk of hemorrhoids and other health conditions associated with prolonged sitting. This can include taking the stairs instead of the elevator, parking further away from the entrance to a building, and taking short breaks throughout the day to stretch or move around.

Natural And Alternative Remedies To Treat Hemorrhoids

While there are many medical treatments available for hemorrhoids, some people prefer natural and alternative remedies. Below we will explore some natural and alternative remedies to treat hemorrhoids.

1. Warm baths: Soaking in a warm bath can help relieve the discomfort of hemorrhoids. Adding Epsom salts or baking soda to the bathwater can also help soothe the affected area.

2. Witch hazel: Witch hazel is a natural astringent that can help reduce swelling and inflammation. Soaking a cotton ball or pad in witch hazel and applying it to the affected area can provide relief.

3. Aloe vera: Aloe vera has anti-inflammatory properties and can help soothe the affected area. Applying aloe vera gel to the affected area can provide relief.

4. Essential oils: Essential oils such as lavender, tea tree, and chamomile can help reduce inflammation and provide pain relief. Diluting a few drops of essential oil in a carrier oil, such as coconut oil, and applying it to the affected area can provide relief.

5. Sitz baths: A sitz bath is a warm, shallow bath that can help soothe the affected area. A sitz bath can be taken in a bathtub or in a special device that fits over the toilet.

6. Dietary changes: Eating a diet high in fiber can help prevent constipation, a common cause of hemorrhoids. Good sources of fiber include fruits, vegetables, whole grains, and legumes.

7. Hydration: Drinking plenty of water can help prevent constipation and dehydration, which can exacerbate hemorrhoids.

8. Exercise: Regular exercise can help improve circulation and prevent constipation, which can help prevent hemorrhoids.

9. Cold compress: Applying a cold compress, such as a cold pack or ice wrapped in a towel, to the affected area can help reduce swelling and provide pain relief.

10. Herbal remedies: Some herbal remedies, such as butcher's broom and horse chestnut, have been shown to be effective in reducing the symptoms of hemorrhoids. It is important to talk to a healthcare provider before using any herbal remedies, as they may interact with other medications or have side effects.

Herbal Treatments, Aloe Vera, Witch Hazel To Treat Hemorrhoids

While there are many medical treatments available for hemorrhoids, some people prefer herbal treatments. Below we will explore two herbal remedies commonly used to treat hemorrhoids: aloe vera and witch hazel.

Aloe vera:

Aloe vera is a succulent plant that is commonly used for medicinal purposes. It has anti-inflammatory and soothing properties and is often used to treat skin conditions such as burns, cuts, and rashes. Aloe vera can also be used to treat hemorrhoids.

To use aloe vera to treat hemorrhoids, the gel from the plant can be applied directly to the affected area. The gel can be extracted by cutting off a leaf from the plant and slicing it open. The gel can be applied to the affected area using a cotton ball or pad. Aloe vera can also be used in the form of a cream or ointment.

Aloe vera has been shown to be effective in reducing the symptoms of hemorrhoids. It can help reduce inflammation and provide relief from pain and itching. Aloe vera is also safe and has few side effects.

Witch hazel:

Witch hazel is a shrub that is native to North America. It has astringent and anti-inflammatory properties and is often used to treat skin conditions such as acne, eczema, and psoriasis. Witch hazel can also be used to treat hemorrhoids.

To use witch hazel to treat hemorrhoids, the liquid extract can be applied to the affected area using a cotton ball or pad. Witch hazel can also be used in the form of a cream or ointment.

Witch hazel has been shown to be effective in reducing the symptoms of hemorrhoids. It can help reduce inflammation and provide relief from pain and itching. Witch hazel is also safe and has few side effects.

Apple Cider Vinegar, Essential Oils, Bioflavonoids

While there are many medical treatments available for hemorrhoids, some people prefer natural remedies. Below we will explore three natural remedies commonly used to treat hemorrhoids: apple cider vinegar, essential oils, and bioflavonoids.

Apple cider vinegar:

Apple cider vinegar is a type of vinegar made from apples. It has antibacterial and anti-inflammatory properties and is often used to treat a variety of conditions, including sore throat, acne, and high cholesterol. Apple cider vinegar can also be used to treat hemorrhoids.

To use apple cider vinegar to treat hemorrhoids, it can be applied to the affected area using a cotton ball or pad. The vinegar should be diluted with water before use, as it can be quite strong. Apple cider vinegar can also be used in the form of a sitz bath.

Apple cider vinegar has been shown to be effective in reducing the symptoms of hemorrhoids. It can help reduce inflammation and provide relief from pain and itching. However, it is important to note that apple cider vinegar can be quite strong and may cause irritation if used in high concentrations.

Essential oils:

Essential oils are concentrated plant extracts that are often used for medicinal purposes. They have a variety of properties, including anti-inflammatory, antibacterial, and analgesic. Essential oils can also be used to treat hemorrhoids.

There are several essential oils that can be used to treat hemorrhoids, including lavender, tea tree, and chamomile. To use essential oils to treat hemorrhoids, they can be diluted in a carrier oil, such as coconut oil, and applied to the affected area using a cotton ball or pad.

Essential oils have been shown to be effective in reducing the symptoms of hemorrhoids. They can help reduce inflammation and provide pain relief. However, it is important to note that essential oils can be quite strong and may cause irritation if used in high concentrations.

Bioflavonoids:

Bioflavonoids are a type of antioxidant that is found in many fruits and vegetables. They have anti-inflammatory properties and are often used to treat conditions such as allergies, arthritis, and high blood pressure. Bioflavonoids can also be used to treat hemorrhoids.

There are several types of bioflavonoids that can be used to treat hemorrhoids, including rutin, hesperidin, and diosmin. Bioflavonoids can be taken in the form of supplements or consumed in foods such as citrus fruits, berries, and leafy green vegetables.

Bioflavonoids have been shown to be effective in reducing the symptoms of hemorrhoids. They can help reduce inflammation and improve blood flow to the affected area. However, it is important to note that bioflavonoids can interact with other medications, so it is important to talk to a healthcare provider before taking supplements.

Chapter Twelve

The role of diet in hemorrhoids

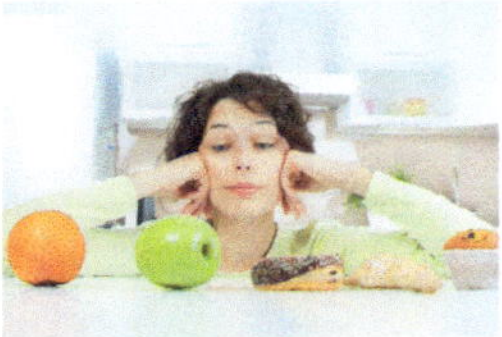

Hemorrhoids, also known as piles, are swollen veins located in the lower rectum and anus. They can be caused by a variety of factors, including genetics, constipation, and straining during bowel movements. However, one factor that plays a significant role in the development of hemorrhoids is diet. In this chapter, we'll explore how different aspects of your diet can affect hemorrhoids and what you can do to prevent and alleviate symptoms.

First and foremost, it's important to understand that a diet high in processed foods and low in fiber can lead to constipation and straining during bowel movements. When you're constipated, you may have to push harder to pass stools, which can put extra pressure on the veins in your rectum and anus. This increased pressure can cause the veins to become swollen and bulge out, leading to hemorrhoids. On the other hand, a diet that is high in fiber can help to prevent constipation by making stools softer and easier to pass. This can reduce the amount of straining you need to do during bowel movements and decrease the risk of developing hemorrhoids.

Fruits, vegetables, whole grains, and legumes are all excellent sources of dietary fiber. Incorporating more of these foods into your diet can help to prevent constipation and reduce the risk of developing hemorrhoids. Additionally, drinking plenty of water can also help to prevent constipation by keeping stools hydrated and soft.

Another dietary factor that can affect hemorrhoids is the consumption of spicy or hot foods. These foods can irritate the sensitive tissues in the rectum and anus, leading to pain, itching, and burning sensations. If you're prone to hemorrhoids, you may want to avoid or limit your intake of spicy foods.

Alcohol and caffeine are also known to dehydrate the body and can cause constipation. If you're prone to hemorrhoids, it may be helpful to reduce your intake of alcohol and caffeine.

Obesity is another risk factor for hemorrhoids. Excess weight can put extra pressure on the veins in the rectum and anus, making it more likely for hemorrhoids to develop. A diet that is high in processed foods and low in fruits, vegetables, and whole grains can contribute to weight gain. Eating a balanced diet that is low in processed foods and high in fiber can help to prevent weight gain and reduce the risk of developing hemorrhoids.

Finally, it's important to note that if you already have hemorrhoids, there are certain foods that you should avoid to alleviate symptoms. These include nuts, seeds, popcorn, and very spicy or hot foods. These foods can irritate the sensitive tissues in the rectum and anus, leading to pain and discomfort.

In conclusion, diet plays a significant role in the development and management of hemorrhoids. A diet high in fiber can help to prevent constipation and reduce the risk of developing hemorrhoids. Additionally, drinking plenty of water, limiting spicy or hot foods, and reducing alcohol and caffeine intake can also be beneficial. Additionally, eating a balanced diet can help to prevent weight gain, which can also contribute to the development of hemorrhoids. If you already have hemorrhoids, certain foods should be avoided to alleviate symptoms. Remember, if you already have hemorrhoids, it is best to consult your doctor for proper diagnosis and treatment.

Chapter Thirteen

The role of stress in hemorrhoids

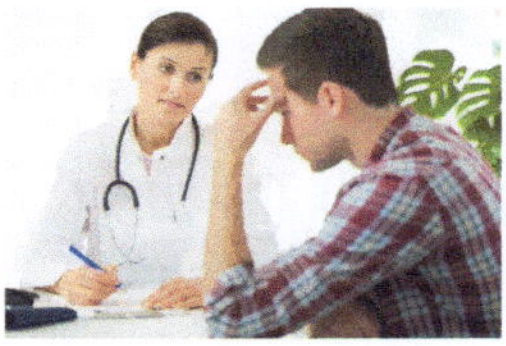

Stress is an inevitable part of our lives. It can come from various sources, such as work, family, or personal issues. While a little bit of stress can be beneficial, as it motivates us to perform at our best, too much stress can be harmful to our physical and mental well-being. One of the many health issues that can be caused by stress is hemorrhoids.

Hemorrhoids, also known as piles, are swollen veins in the lower rectum and anus. They can be caused by a variety of factors, such as obesity, pregnancy, and constipation. However, stress also plays a significant role in the development of hemorrhoids.

When we are stressed, our body goes into a "fight or flight" mode. This causes an increase in the levels of adrenaline and cortisol, two hormones that are responsible for the body's response to stress. These hormones cause the blood vessels in the rectum and anus to dilate, leading to inflammation and swelling of the veins.

Additionally, stress can also lead to an increase in the muscle tone of the anal sphincter, the muscle that controls the opening and closing of the anus. This can cause difficulty in passing stools, leading to constipation, which is another common cause of hemorrhoids.

Apart from the physical effects of stress on hemorrhoids, there is also a psychological aspect to it. Stress can cause anxiety and depression, which can lead to a change in bowel habits. People who are stressed may hold in their stools, leading to constipation and hemorrhoids.

In addition, stress can also lead to an increase in the consumption of certain foods and drinks that are known to cause hemorrhoids. For example, people who are stressed may turn to foods that are high in fat and sugar, as well as alcohol and caffeine, which can cause dehydration and constipation, leading to hemorrhoids.

To prevent hemorrhoids caused by stress, it is important to manage stress levels. This can be done by practicing stress-relieving activities such as yoga, meditation, and regular exercise.

Eating a healthy and balanced diet, rich in fruits and vegetables, and drinking enough water can also prevent constipation and hemorrhoids.

In addition, if you have a sedentary job, try to get up and move around every hour, to get the blood flowing.

In the event that you already have hemorrhoids, it is important to avoid activities that can worsen them such as heavy lifting, long periods of standing or sitting, and straining during bowel movements.

If your hemorrhoids are particularly severe or if home treatment methods are not working, it's best to visit a doctor who may be able to provide you with more specific treatment options such as medication, procedures or surgery.

In conclusion, stress plays a significant role in the development of hemorrhoids. By managing stress levels, eating a healthy diet and avoiding activities that can worsen hemorrhoids, you can prevent and treat this condition. It's always best to consult with a medical professional if you are experiencing symptoms of hemorrhoids or have any other concerns about your health.

Chapter Fourteen

What are the risks and complications associated with hemorrhoids?

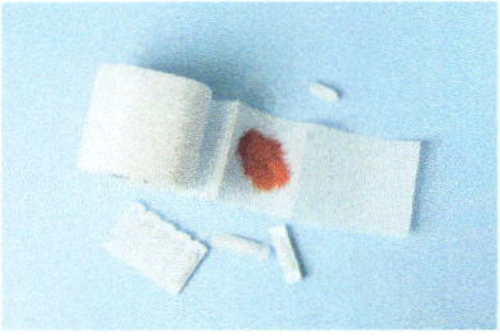

Hemorrhoids, also known as piles, are a common ailment that affects the rectum and anus. They occur when the veins in these areas become swollen and inflamed, which can lead to a variety of symptoms such as itching, pain, and bleeding. While hemorrhoids are generally not a serious condition, they can be quite uncomfortable and can even lead to more serious complications if left untreated.

One of the most common complications associated with hemorrhoids is bleeding. This can occur when the swollen veins in the rectum and anus rupture, leading to the release of blood. This bleeding can be quite heavy at times and may require medical attention. In some cases, the bleeding may be caused by a more serious condition, such as a tumor, and may require further investigation to determine the underlying cause.

Another common complication associated with hemorrhoids is thrombosis. This occurs when a blood clot forms within the swollen vein, leading to severe pain and inflammation. Thrombosis can be quite dangerous, as the blood clot can break off and travel to the lungs, causing a potentially fatal condition known as a pulmonary embolism.

Another risk associated with hemorrhoids is that of infection. The rectum and anus are home to a variety of bacteria, and these can easily infect the swollen veins of the hemorrhoids. This can lead to an abscess, which is a pocket of pus that forms in the tissue around the anus. Abscesses can be quite painful and can even lead to fever and chills if the infection spreads.

Prolapse is another risk associated with hemorrhoids. This occurs when the hemorrhoid becomes so swollen that it protrudes from the anus. This can be quite uncomfortable and can also lead to further complications such as bleeding, thrombosis, and infection. In some cases, surgery may be required to correct a prolapsed hemorrhoid.

Another complication associated with hemorrhoids is fecal incontinence. This occurs when the hemorrhoids become so swollen that they block the normal passage of feces. This can lead to difficulty passing bowel movements and can also lead to leakage of feces.

Finally, hemorrhoids can lead to itching and discomfort around the anus. This can be quite distracting and can make it difficult to focus on daily tasks. The itching can be caused by the inflammation of the hemorrhoids, as well as by the presence of bacteria in the area.

In conclusion, hemorrhoids are a common ailment that can lead to a variety of complications if left untreated. These complications can include bleeding, thrombosis, infection, prolapse, fecal incontinence, and itching and discomfort around the anus. If you suspect that you may have hemorrhoids, it is important to see a doctor for an examination and treatment. There are many different treatment options available, including lifestyle changes, over-the-counter medications, and surgery, so it is important to find the right treatment plan for you.

Complications And Risks Associated With Hemorrhoids

While hemorrhoids are typically not a serious health condition, they can lead to complications and risks if left untreated. Below we will explore the complications and risks associated with hemorrhoids.

Complications of Hemorrhoids:

- Thrombosis: Thrombosis occurs when a blood clot forms in a hemorrhoid, leading to severe pain and discomfort. Thrombosed hemorrhoids can be treated with a variety of methods, including excision or ligation.

- Anemia: Chronic bleeding from hemorrhoids can lead to anemia, a condition characterized by a low red blood cell count. Anemia can lead to fatigue, weakness, and shortness of breath.

- Strangulation: Strangulation occurs when a hemorrhoid becomes trapped outside of the anus and the blood supply is cut off. Strangulated hemorrhoids can be a medical emergency and require immediate treatment.

- Infection: Hemorrhoids can become infected, leading to pain, swelling, and discharge. Infection can be treated with antibiotics, but may require drainage in some cases.

- Fistula: A fistula is an abnormal connection between the anus or rectum and another area of the body, such as the vagina or bladder. Fistulas can occur as a complication of hemorrhoids and require surgical treatment.

Risks of Hemorrhoids:

- Recurrence: Hemorrhoids can recur, especially if the underlying cause of the hemorrhoids is not addressed. Recurrent hemorrhoids may require more aggressive treatment, such as surgery.
- Chronic pain: Chronic pain can occur as a result of hemorrhoids, particularly if the hemorrhoids become chronic or recurrent. Chronic pain can significantly impact quality of life and require ongoing management.
- Impaired quality of life: Hemorrhoids can significantly impair quality of life, leading to embarrassment, anxiety, and avoidance of social situations. Hemorrhoids can also impact sexual function and lead to relationship problems.
- Colon cancer: While the risk of colon cancer is not directly related to hemorrhoids, chronic bleeding from hemorrhoids can mask the symptoms of colon cancer. It is important to seek medical attention if you are experiencing chronic bleeding from hemorrhoids or any other symptoms of colon cancer.
- Incontinence: In rare cases, hemorrhoid surgery can lead to damage to the muscles that control bowel function, leading to incontinence. This is a rare complication, but it is important to discuss the risks and benefits of hemorrhoid surgery with a healthcare provider.

Anemia, Infection, Thrombosis, Strangulated Hemorrhoids, Rectal Prolapse

While hemorrhoids are typically not a serious health condition, they can lead to complications and risks if left untreated. Below we will explore several complications of hemorrhoids, including anemia, infection, thrombosis, strangulated hemorrhoids, and rectal prolapse.

Anemia:

Anemia is a condition characterized by a low red blood cell count. Chronic bleeding from hemorrhoids can lead to anemia, as blood loss leads to a decreased number of red blood cells in the body. Symptoms of anemia include fatigue, weakness, and shortness of breath. Treatment for anemia typically involves iron supplements or, in severe cases, blood transfusions.

Infection:

Hemorrhoids can become infected, leading to pain, swelling, and discharge. Infection can occur when bacteria enter the area around the hemorrhoid, typically through a break in the skin or mucous membrane. Infection can be treated with antibiotics, but may require drainage in some cases.

Thrombosis:

Thrombosis occurs when a blood clot forms in a hemorrhoid, leading to severe pain and discomfort. Thrombosed hemorrhoids can be treated with a variety of methods, including excision or ligation. Treatment for thrombosed hemorrhoids typically involves a combination of pain management and surgical intervention.

Strangulated Hemorrhoids:

Strangulation occurs when a hemorrhoid becomes trapped outside of the anus and the blood supply is cut off. Strangulated hemorrhoids can be a medical emergency and require immediate treatment. Symptoms of strangulated hemorrhoids include severe pain, swelling, and the presence of a blue or purple lump around the anus. Treatment for strangulated hemorrhoids typically involves surgical intervention.

Rectal Prolapse:

Rectal prolapse is a condition in which the rectum protrudes from the anus. Prolapse can occur as a complication of hemorrhoids, particularly in cases where the hemorrhoids are chronic or recurrent. Symptoms of rectal prolapse include the sensation of a lump around the anus, difficulty passing stool, and fecal incontinence. Treatment for rectal prolapse typically involves surgical intervention.

Chapter Fifteen

Living with hemorrhoids

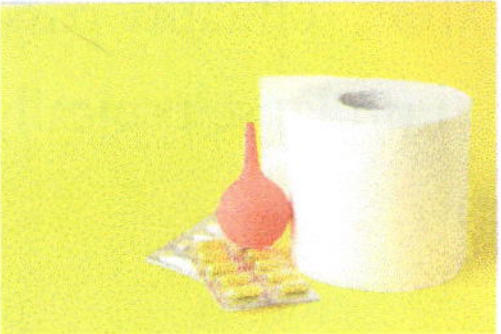

Living with hemorrhoids can be uncomfortable and embarrassing, but with the right treatment and lifestyle changes, it is possible to manage the symptoms and improve your quality of life.

One of the most important things you can do to manage hemorrhoids is to maintain a healthy diet. Eating a diet high in fiber can help to reduce constipation and relieve pressure in the lower rectum. Good sources of fiber include fruits, vegetables, whole grains, and legumes. Drinking plenty of water can also help to keep stools soft and prevent constipation.

Another important aspect of living with hemorrhoids is to maintain good bathroom habits. Try to avoid straining during bowel movements, and don't spend too much time on the toilet. If you are experiencing constipation, try to avoid using laxatives, as they can cause diarrhea and make hemorrhoids worse. Instead, try to increase your fiber and water intake to encourage regular bowel movements.

Exercise is also an important aspect of managing hemorrhoids. Regular physical activity can help to reduce constipation, relieve pressure in the lower rectum, and improve circulation. Aim for at least 30 minutes of moderate-intensity exercise, such as brisk walking, jogging, cycling, or swimming, most days of the week.

If you are experiencing symptoms such as itching, burning, or pain, there are several over-the-counter creams, ointments, and suppositories that can provide relief. Be sure to follow the instructions on the label, and avoid using these products for more than a week at a time. If symptoms persist, it is important to see your doctor for a proper diagnosis and treatment plan.

In some cases, your doctor may recommend one of several medical procedures to treat hemorrhoids. Rubber band ligation is a common procedure that involves placing a small rubber band around the base of the hemorrhoid to cut off its blood supply, causing it to shrink and eventually fall off. Sclerotherapy is another procedure that involves injecting a solution into the hemorrhoid to shrink it.

In severe cases, surgery may be necessary to remove the hemorrhoids. The surgery is called hemorrhoidectomy. This is typically done under general anesthesia and involves removing the hemorrhoids and the surrounding tissue. Recovery from surgery can take several weeks and may include pain, bleeding, and difficulty with bowel movements.

Living with hemorrhoids can be challenging, but it is important to remember that there are many treatment options available. With the right treatment and lifestyle changes, it is possible to manage the symptoms and improve your quality of life.

It's also important to note that, having hemorrhoids does not mean that you have to compromise your lifestyle. You can still continue to do the things you love like going to the gym, going for a swim or even cycling. However, it's important to pay attention to any discomfort or pain you might experience and to adjust your workout routine accordingly.

It's also important to remember that hemorrhoids are a common condition, and there's no need to feel embarrassed or ashamed about them. Many people experience hemorrhoids at some point in their lives, and there are many treatment options available to help manage the symptoms. If you're experiencing symptoms, it's important to see your doctor for a proper diagnosis and treatment plan.

In addition, there are several things you can do at home to help relieve symptoms of hemorrhoids. For example, sitz baths, which involve sitting in warm water for 10-15 minutes, can help to relieve itching, burning, and pain. Applying a cold compress, such as a bag of frozen peas or a cold gel pack, to the area can also help to reduce inflammation and provide relief.

Hemorrhoids And Mental Health

While the physical symptoms of hemorrhoids can be uncomfortable and painful, they can also have an impact on mental health.

One of the main ways that hemorrhoids can impact mental health is through the physical discomfort and pain that they cause. Hemorrhoids can cause itching, burning, and pain, which can be difficult to manage and can lead to feelings of frustration, irritability, and anxiety. The constant discomfort can also impact sleep, which can lead to feelings of fatigue and exhaustion.

In addition to the physical discomfort, hemorrhoids can also impact mental health through their impact on daily activities. Hemorrhoids can make it difficult to sit for long periods of time, which can impact work, socializing, and other daily activities. This can lead to feelings of isolation and loneliness, as well as feelings of inadequacy and frustration.

Hemorrhoids can also impact mental health through the stigma associated with the condition. Hemorrhoids are often seen as embarrassing and shameful, which can lead to feelings of self-consciousness and low self-esteem. This can impact relationships, work, and other aspects of life, and can lead to feelings of depression and anxiety.

The impact of hemorrhoids on mental health is not just limited to the physical symptoms and stigma associated with the condition. The treatment of hemorrhoids can also impact mental health. Some treatments, such as surgery, can be invasive and can require a long recovery time. This can impact work, socializing, and other aspects of life, and can lead to feelings of frustration and isolation.

It is important to address the impact of hemorrhoids on mental health. There are several ways to manage the mental health impact of hemorrhoids, including:

1. Talking to a healthcare provider about treatment options: There are many treatment options available for hemorrhoids, and it is important to find the right treatment for you. Talking to a healthcare provider can help you find a treatment that is effective and minimally invasive.

2. Seeking support: It is important to have a support system when dealing with any medical condition. This can include family, friends, and support groups. Talking to others who have experienced hemorrhoids can help you feel less alone and can provide valuable advice and support.

3. Practicing self-care: Self-care is important for both physical and mental health. This can include activities such as exercise, meditation, and relaxation techniques. Taking time for yourself can help reduce stress and improve mental health.

4. Seeking professional help: If you are experiencing symptoms of depression or anxiety related to hemorrhoids, it may be helpful to seek professional help. A therapist or counselor can provide support and guidance for managing the mental health impact of hemorrhoids.

The Impact Of Hemorrhoids On Mental Well-Being

Hemorrhoids are a common medical condition that can cause discomfort, pain, and bleeding. While the physical symptoms of hemorrhoids are well-known, the impact of this condition on mental well-being is often overlooked. The discomfort and pain associated with hemorrhoids can have a significant impact on a person's mental health, causing stress, anxiety, and depression. Below we will explore the impact of hemorrhoids on mental well-being and the strategies that can be used to manage this impact.

Physical pain and discomfort caused by hemorrhoids can lead to feelings of stress and anxiety. People may become concerned about the pain and discomfort that they experience, which can lead to a sense of uncertainty and worry about their future health. This can cause them to feel stressed and anxious, which can negatively impact their mental health.

In addition, the pain and discomfort caused by hemorrhoids can make it difficult for people to perform daily tasks such as sitting, walking, and standing for long periods of time. This can cause feelings of frustration and helplessness, leading to a sense of hopelessness and depression.

Hemorrhoids can also lead to feelings of embarrassment and shame. Many people feel embarrassed about discussing the condition with their doctor or loved ones, which can lead to a sense of isolation and loneliness. This can further worsen their mental well-being and lead to negative thoughts and feelings.

Furthermore, the financial burden of treating hemorrhoids can also impact mental well-being. The cost of medications, procedures, and surgeries can be expensive, which can cause financial stress and anxiety.

However, there are several strategies that can be used to manage the impact of hemorrhoids on mental well-being. These include:

1. Seeking medical help: The first step in managing the impact of hemorrhoids on mental well-being is to seek medical help. A healthcare provider can recommend treatments that can help relieve the pain and discomfort associated with hemorrhoids. They can also offer advice on lifestyle changes that can help prevent hemorrhoids from occurring in the future.

2. Practicing self-care: Practicing self-care is essential for maintaining good mental health. People can engage in activities such as meditation, deep breathing, yoga, and exercise to help reduce stress and anxiety.

3. Seeking social support: Talking to friends, family, or a support group can help individuals feel less isolated and more supported. This can provide a sense of comfort and help alleviate negative thoughts and feelings.

4. Cognitive-behavioral therapy: Cognitive-behavioral therapy (CBT) is a type of therapy that can help individuals manage the negative thoughts and feelings associated with hemorrhoids. This therapy focuses on changing negative thought patterns and developing coping strategies to manage stress and anxiety.

Dealing With Embarrassment And Stigma

Hemorrhoids are a common medical condition that affects millions of people worldwide. Despite their prevalence, hemorrhoids are often stigmatized, and many people feel embarrassed or ashamed to discuss the condition with others. This stigma can make it difficult for people to seek treatment, and it can impact their mental health and quality of life. Below we will discuss how to deal with embarrassment and stigma associated with hemorrhoids.

One of the main challenges of dealing with embarrassment and stigma associated with hemorrhoids is overcoming the societal taboos that surround the condition. Many people feel embarrassed to discuss hemorrhoids with others, even their healthcare provider, because they view the condition as private or shameful. This can make it difficult to seek treatment, and it can also prevent individuals from discussing their symptoms with family and friends.

To overcome this challenge, it is important to recognize that hemorrhoids are a common medical condition that affects many people. Discussing the condition with a healthcare provider can help individuals understand that they are not alone, and that there are effective treatments available.

Another way to overcome embarrassment and stigma associated with hemorrhoids is to educate oneself about the condition. Learning about the causes, symptoms, and treatments of hemorrhoids can help individuals feel more empowered and confident when discussing the condition with others.

Furthermore, it is important to remember that hemorrhoids are a medical condition, and that seeking treatment is a normal and necessary part of managing the condition. Rather than feeling ashamed or embarrassed, individuals should focus on taking care of their health and well-being.

Another strategy for dealing with embarrassment and stigma associated with hemorrhoids is to seek support from others. Talking to friends or family members who have experienced hemorrhoids can provide valuable support and advice. Additionally, joining a support group for individuals with hemorrhoids can provide a sense of community and reduce feelings of isolation.

In addition to seeking support from others, it is important to practice self-compassion and self-care. This can include engaging in activities that promote relaxation, such as meditation or yoga, and taking time for oneself to engage in enjoyable activities.

Finally, it is important to remember that everyone experiences health challenges at some point in their lives. Rather than feeling embarrassed or ashamed, individuals with hemorrhoids should focus on taking care of themselves and managing their symptoms.

Building A Support System

Living with a medical condition such as hemorrhoids can be challenging and overwhelming. One of the most important things that individuals can do to manage the condition and improve their overall well-being is to build a support system. A support system can provide emotional support, practical assistance, and a sense of community, all of which are essential for coping with the challenges of living with hemorrhoids. Below we will discuss the benefits of building a support system and strategies for doing so.

Benefits of Building a Support System

Building a support system can have numerous benefits for individuals living with hemorrhoids. Some of the key benefits include:

1. Emotional Support: A support system can provide emotional support, which can help individuals cope with the stress and anxiety associated with the condition. Emotional support can come in the form of listening, empathy, and understanding.

2. Practical Assistance: A support system can also provide practical assistance, such as help with daily tasks, transportation to medical appointments, and financial assistance. This can help individuals manage the practical challenges of living with hemorrhoids.

3. Sense of Community: Building a support system can also provide a sense of community and belonging, which can reduce feelings of isolation and loneliness.

Strategies for Building a Support System

Building a support system can seem daunting, but there are several strategies that individuals can use to create a supportive network. These strategies include:

4. Reach Out to Family and Friends: One of the simplest ways to build a support system is to reach out to family and friends. This can include discussing the condition with loved ones, seeking their support and assistance, and engaging in activities that promote social connection.

5. Join a Support Group: Joining a support group for individuals with hemorrhoids can provide a sense of community and connection with others who are experiencing similar challenges. Support groups can be found through online resources, healthcare providers, or community organizations.

6. Seek Professional Help: Seeking professional help from a healthcare provider, therapist, or counselor can also provide emotional support and practical assistance for managing the condition.

7. Practice Self-Care: Practicing self-care can also be an important part of building a support system. This can include engaging in activities that promote relaxation and stress reduction, such as meditation or exercise.

8. Utilize Online Resources: Online resources such as forums, blogs, and social media groups can provide a sense of community and connection with others who are living with hemorrhoids. These resources can also provide information and advice for managing the condition.

Seeking Professional Help When Necessary

Hemorrhoids are a common medical condition that can be managed with self-care and over-the-counter treatments in many cases. However, in some cases, seeking professional help may be necessary. This can include consultation with a healthcare provider, therapist, or specialist. Below we will discuss the importance of seeking professional help when necessary and strategies for doing so.

Why Seek Professional Help?

Seeking professional help can be important for several reasons. For example:

1. Accurate Diagnosis: A healthcare provider can provide an accurate diagnosis of the condition and determine the appropriate course of treatment. In some cases, symptoms that may appear to be hemorrhoids could be indicative of a more serious condition, such as colorectal cancer.

2. Access to Medical Treatments: A healthcare provider can also provide access to medical treatments that may not be available over-the-counter. This can include prescription medications, minimally invasive procedures, and surgical interventions.

3. Emotional Support: In addition to medical treatment, seeking professional help can also provide emotional support for individuals who may be struggling with the emotional toll of living with hemorrhoids.

Strategies for Seeking Professional Help

Seeking professional help can seem daunting, but there are several strategies that individuals can use to make the process easier:

4. Research Healthcare Providers: Researching healthcare providers in the local area can be a good place to start. This can include reading reviews online, asking for referrals from friends or family members, or contacting local healthcare organizations.

5. Schedule an Appointment: Once a healthcare provider is identified, schedule an appointment to discuss symptoms and treatment options. Be prepared to provide a detailed medical history and description of symptoms.

6. Ask Questions: It is important to ask questions during the appointment to ensure that all concerns are addressed. This can include questions about treatment options, potential risks and side effects, and any other concerns related to the condition.

7. Consider a Second Opinion: If there is any doubt about the diagnosis or treatment plan, consider seeking a second opinion from another healthcare provider.

8. Seek Support: If emotional support is needed, consider seeking support from a therapist or counselor. These professionals can provide a safe and confidential space to discuss feelings and concerns related to the condition.

Seeking professional help can be an important part of managing hemorrhoids. A healthcare provider can provide an accurate diagnosis, access to medical treatments, and emotional support. Strategies for seeking professional help include researching healthcare providers, scheduling an appointment, asking questions, considering a second opinion, and seeking support from a therapist or counselor. By taking these steps, individuals can better manage the condition and improve their overall well-being.

Conclusion: Living With Hemorrhoids

Living with hemorrhoids can be challenging, but it is important to understand that there are effective treatments and management strategies available. By seeking out accurate information, working with healthcare providers, and implementing preventative measures, individuals can manage their symptoms effectively and improve their quality of life.

It is important to seek medical advice if you have hemorrhoids, as they can lead to complications such as anemia, infection, thrombosis, strangulated hemorrhoids, and rectal prolapse. Accurate diagnosis and treatment can prevent these complications and ensure that individuals receive appropriate care.

Individuals can also take preventative measures to reduce their risk of developing hemorrhoids. This includes maintaining a healthy weight, staying hydrated, increasing fiber intake, and avoiding constipation. Regular exercise, maintaining healthy bowel habits, and avoiding prolonged sitting can also help prevent hemorrhoids.

Effective treatments for hemorrhoids include topical medications, oral medications, sclerotherapy, rubber band ligation, infrared coagulation, and surgery. The choice of treatment will depend on the severity of symptoms and the individual's unique needs and circumstances.

Living with hemorrhoids can also impact an individual's mental well-being, as the condition can be embarrassing and stigmatized. Building a support system and seeking professional help if necessary can help individuals manage their emotional well-being and improve their quality of life.

Living with hemorrhoids can be challenging, but there are effective treatments and management strategies available. By seeking out accurate information, working with healthcare providers, implementing preventative measures, and managing their emotional well-being, individuals can manage their symptoms effectively and improve their quality of life. It is essential to seek medical advice if you have hemorrhoids and to challenge myths and misconceptions about the condition to promote accurate knowledge and prevent misunderstandings.

Overcoming The Challenges Of Hemorrhoids

Hemorrhoids can be a challenging condition to manage, as they can cause discomfort, pain, and embarrassment. However, by implementing effective strategies and seeking out appropriate treatments, individuals can overcome the challenges of hemorrhoids and improve their quality of life. Below we will explore strategies for overcoming the challenges of hemorrhoids.

Seek Medical Advice

One of the most important strategies for overcoming the challenges of hemorrhoids is to seek medical advice. Healthcare providers can provide accurate diagnoses, recommend appropriate treatments, and monitor symptoms to ensure that individuals receive the best care possible. By seeking medical advice, individuals can ensure that their symptoms are properly managed and prevent complications.

Implement Preventative Measures

Implementing preventative measures is another important strategy for overcoming the challenges of hemorrhoids. This includes maintaining healthy bowel habits, increasing fiber intake, staying hydrated, and avoiding constipation. Regular exercise, avoiding prolonged sitting, and maintaining a healthy weight can also help prevent hemorrhoids.

Use Effective Treatments

Effective treatments are essential for overcoming the challenges of hemorrhoids. Topical medications, oral medications, sclerotherapy, rubber band ligation, infrared coagulation, and surgery are all effective treatment options for hemorrhoids. The choice of treatment will depend on the severity of symptoms and the individual's unique needs and circumstances.

Manage Emotional Well-Being

Living with hemorrhoids can impact an individual's emotional well-being, as the condition can be embarrassing and stigmatized. Building a support system, seeking professional help if necessary, and challenging myths and misconceptions about hemorrhoids can help individuals manage their emotional well-being and improve their quality of life.

Practice Self-Care

Practicing self-care is also important for overcoming the challenges of hemorrhoids. This includes taking time for oneself, engaging in activities that bring joy and fulfillment, and managing stress levels. By practicing self-care, individuals can reduce the impact of hemorrhoids on their overall well-being.

Overcoming the challenges of hemorrhoids requires a multi-faceted approach. By seeking medical advice, implementing preventative measures, using effective treatments, managing emotional well-being, and practicing self-care, individuals can manage their symptoms effectively and improve their quality of life. It is important to challenge myths and misconceptions about hemorrhoids, seek appropriate care, and take steps to prevent the condition from occurring in the first place. By doing so, individuals can live healthy, fulfilling lives and overcome the challenges of hemorrhoids.

Finding The Right Treatment Plan

Finding the right treatment plan for hemorrhoids can be challenging, as there are various treatment options available. However, by working with healthcare providers, understanding the different treatment options, and considering individual needs and circumstances, individuals can find the right treatment plan for their unique needs. Below we will explore strategies for finding the right treatment plan for hemorrhoids.

Seek Medical Advice

One of the most important strategies for finding the right treatment plan for hemorrhoids is to seek medical advice. Healthcare providers can provide accurate diagnoses, recommend appropriate treatments, and monitor symptoms to ensure that individuals receive the best care possible. By seeking medical advice, individuals can ensure that their symptoms are properly managed and prevent complications.

Understand Different Treatment Options

Another important strategy for finding the right treatment plan for hemorrhoids is to understand the different treatment options. Topical medications, oral medications, sclerotherapy, rubber band ligation, infrared coagulation, and surgery are all effective treatment options for hemorrhoids. Understanding the pros and cons of each treatment option can help individuals make informed decisions about their care.

Consider Individual Needs and Circumstances

Individual needs and circumstances should also be considered when finding the right treatment plan for hemorrhoids. This includes factors such as the severity of symptoms, the individual's overall health, and any other medical conditions or medications. By considering individual needs and circumstances, healthcare providers can recommend the most appropriate treatment plan for each individual.

Evaluate Risks and Benefits

Evaluating the risks and benefits of each treatment option is also important for finding the right treatment plan for hemorrhoids. Some treatment options may have more significant risks or side effects than others, while some may be more effective at managing symptoms. By evaluating the risks and benefits, individuals can make informed decisions about their care.

Work with Healthcare Providers

Working with healthcare providers is crucial for finding the right treatment plan for hemorrhoids. Healthcare providers can provide valuable insights and recommendations, monitor symptoms, and adjust treatment plans as necessary. By working with healthcare providers, individuals can ensure that their care is tailored to their unique needs and circumstances.

Finding the right treatment plan for hemorrhoids requires a multi-faceted approach. By seeking medical advice, understanding the different treatment options, considering individual needs and circumstances, evaluating risks and benefits, and working with healthcare providers, individuals can find the right treatment plan for their unique needs. It is essential to seek appropriate care, challenge myths and misconceptions about hemorrhoids, and take steps to prevent the condition from occurring in the first place. By doing so, individuals can manage their symptoms effectively and improve their quality of life.

Embracing A Healthier Lifestyle Hemorrhoids

Embracing a healthier lifestyle is an important strategy for managing hemorrhoids and preventing them from occurring in the first place. By adopting healthy habits, individuals can reduce their risk of developing hemorrhoids and manage their symptoms more effectively. Below we will explore strategies for embracing a healthier lifestyle to manage hemorrhoids.

Increase Fiber Intake

One of the most important strategies for embracing a healthier lifestyle to manage hemorrhoids is to increase fiber intake. Fiber helps to soften stool, making it easier to pass, and reduces the risk of constipation. Good sources of fiber include whole grains, fruits, vegetables, and legumes.

Stay Hydrated

Staying hydrated is also important for managing hemorrhoids. Drinking plenty of water and other fluids can help prevent constipation and soften stool. It is recommended that individuals drink at least eight glasses of water per day.

Regular Exercise

Regular exercise is essential for maintaining good health and managing hemorrhoids. Exercise helps to promote bowel regularity and reduces the risk of constipation. It also helps to reduce stress levels, which can worsen hemorrhoid symptoms.

Avoid Prolonged Sitting

Avoiding prolonged sitting is another important strategy for managing hemorrhoids. Sitting for long periods can increase pressure on the rectal area, which can worsen hemorrhoid symptoms. Taking breaks and standing up and stretching can help reduce pressure and prevent symptoms from occurring.

Maintain Healthy Bowel Habits

Maintaining healthy bowel habits is essential for managing hemorrhoids. This includes going to the bathroom when the urge arises, avoiding straining during bowel movements, and not delaying bowel movements. It is also important to use gentle wipes or wet toilet paper instead of dry toilet paper, as dry toilet paper can irritate the rectal area.

Manage Stress

Managing stress levels is also important for managing hemorrhoids. Stress can worsen hemorrhoid symptoms and lead to increased inflammation in the body. Engaging in stress-reducing activities such as meditation, yoga, or deep breathing exercises can help manage stress levels and improve overall well-being.

Embracing a healthier lifestyle is an important strategy for managing hemorrhoids and preventing them from occurring in the first place. Increasing fiber intake, staying hydrated, regular exercise, avoiding prolonged sitting, maintaining healthy bowel habits, and managing stress levels are all effective strategies for managing hemorrhoids. It is important to seek medical advice if hemorrhoid symptoms persist or worsen, and to challenge myths and misconceptions about hemorrhoids to promote accurate knowledge and understanding. By adopting healthy habits, individuals can manage their symptoms effectively and improve their quality of life.

The Importance Of Self-Care And Support To Treat Hemorrhoids

Self-care and support are essential for treating hemorrhoids and managing the symptoms associated with this condition. Hemorrhoids can be a painful and uncomfortable condition, and it can be challenging to manage symptoms alone. Below we will explore the importance of self-care and support for treating hemorrhoids.

Practice Good Hygiene

Practicing good hygiene is essential for treating hemorrhoids. It is important to keep the anal area clean and dry to prevent irritation and reduce the risk of infection. After bowel movements, it is recommended to use a gentle wipe or wet toilet paper, followed by patting dry with a clean towel.

Use Topical Medications

Topical medications such as creams and ointments can help reduce inflammation, relieve pain and itching, and shrink hemorrhoids. These medications are available over-the-counter or by prescription and can be an effective treatment option for managing symptoms.

Seek Professional Help

Seeking professional help is essential for managing hemorrhoids. Healthcare providers can provide accurate diagnoses, recommend appropriate treatments, and monitor symptoms to ensure that individuals receive the best care possible. By seeking medical advice, individuals can ensure that their symptoms are properly managed and prevent complications.

Practice Stress-Reduction Techniques

Stress can worsen hemorrhoid symptoms, so it is essential to practice stress-reduction techniques such as meditation, yoga, or deep breathing exercises. Engaging in these activities can help manage stress levels and improve overall well-being.

Find a Support System

Having a support system can be crucial for managing hemorrhoids. Family members, friends, or support groups can provide emotional support, help with daily tasks, and assist in finding appropriate medical care. Having a support system can also reduce feelings of isolation and improve overall well-being.

Practice Self-Care

Practicing self-care is essential for managing hemorrhoids. This includes getting enough sleep, eating a healthy diet, engaging in physical activity, and taking time for self-care activities such as reading, taking a bath, or practicing a hobby. Taking care of oneself can improve overall well-being and reduce stress levels.

Self-care and support are essential for treating hemorrhoids and managing the associated symptoms. Practicing good hygiene, using topical medications, seeking professional help, practicing stress-reduction techniques, finding a support system, and practicing self-care are all effective strategies for managing hemorrhoids. It is important to seek appropriate care, challenge myths and misconceptions about hemorrhoids, and take steps to prevent the condition from occurring in the first place. By doing so, individuals can manage their symptoms effectively and improve their quality of life.

Chapter Sixteen

FAQ

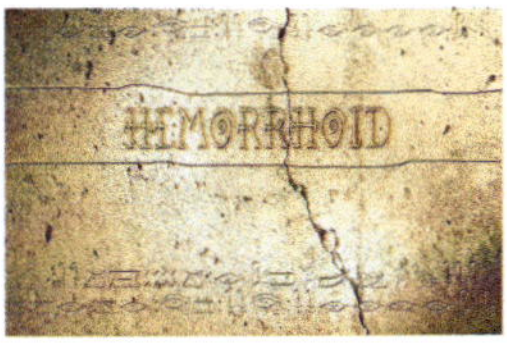

How do I get rid of my hemorrhoids?

There is no one definitive answer to the question of how to get rid of hemorrhoids. Some people find that home remedies, such as changes in diet and increased hydration, are effective in relieving symptoms. Others may need to try over-the-counter or prescription medications. In some cases, surgery may be necessary to remove hemorrhoids.

Individuals with hemorrhoids may experience symptoms such as anal itching, pain, or bleeding. Bleeding from hemorrhoids often occurs during bowel movements, and blood may be visible on toilet paper or in the toilet bowl. Hemorrhoids can be uncomfortable and painful, but they usually do not require medical treatment.

There are a number of home remedies that may help to relieve symptoms. These include:

- Eating a high-fiber diet. This helps to soften stool and reduce strain during bowel movements.

- Drinking plenty of fluids. This helps to keep the stool hydrated and soft.

- Avoiding constipation and diarrhea.

- Taking over-the-counter stool softeners or fiber supplements.

- Applying over-the-counter topical creams or ointments.

- Soaking the anal area in warm water for 10-15 minutes several times a day.

If home remedies do not improve symptoms, there are several over-the-counter medications that may be effective. These include:

- Hemorrhoid creams or ointments that contain a local anesthetic. This can help to numb the area and relieve pain.

- Creams or ointments that contain steroids. These can help to reduce inflammation.

- Hemorrhoid pads that contain Witch Hazel or a similar ingredient. This can help to soothe and reduce swelling.

If over-the-counter treatments do not improve symptoms, a doctor may prescribe a stronger medication. These include:

- Corticosteroid creams or ointments.

- Prescription-strength stool softeners.

- Antibiotic ointments, if there is evidence of infection.

In some cases, surgery may be necessary to remove hemorrhoids. This is generally only recommended for severe cases that do not respond to other treatments. Surgery is typically a last resort option.

Do hemorrhoids go away on its own?

Hemorrhoids are a common condition that affects millions of people each year. While hemorrhoids often resolve on their own, sometimes they can become a chronic problem.

There are two types of hemorrhoids: internal and external. Internal hemorrhoids are located inside the rectum, while external hemorrhoids are located under the skin around the anus. Hemorrhoids are usually caused by increased pressure in the anal or rectal area. This pressure can be due to pregnancy, constipation, diarrhea, or even extended periods of sitting.

While hemorrhoids often go away on their own, sometimes they can become a chronic problem. Chronic hemorrhoids can be quite painful and may require treatment. Treatment options for hemorrhoids include over-the-counter creams and ointments, stool softeners, ice packs, sitz baths, and surgery.

If you have hemorrhoids, be sure to talk to your doctor. They can help you determine the best course of treatment.

How do u know if u have a hemorrhoid?

There are a few different ways to find out if you have hemorrhoids. The most common way is to look for symptoms like bleeding during a bowel movement, itching or irritation in the anal area, or pain or discomfort when sitting or standing for long periods of time.

Another way to tell if you have hemorrhoids is to have a doctor or other medical professional check for them. This can be done during a digital rectal exam, where the doctor inserts a gloved, lubricated finger into the rectum to feel for hemorrhoids.

Yet another way to determine if you have hemorrhoids is to look for them during a colonoscopy or sigmoidoscopy. These procedures involve inserting a small camera into the rectum and colon to look for abnormal growths, including hemorrhoids.

If you think you might have hemorrhoids, it's important to see a doctor so they can rule out other potential causes of your symptoms, like anal fissures, anal fistulas, or rectal prolapse.

Are hemorrhoids a serious thing?

Hemorrhoids are a very common problem, affecting up to one third of the population. They most often occur in people between the ages of 20 and 50.

There are two types of hemorrhoids: internal and external. Internal hemorrhoids are located inside the rectum. They are usually not painful but can bleed. External hemorrhoids are located under the skin around the anus. They can be painful and often bleed.

Hemorrhoids are not a serious medical problem but can be a very uncomfortable one. They are usually treated with over-the-counter creams, ointments, and suppositories. In some cases, surgery may be necessary.

What happens if hemorrhoids go untreated?

If hemorrhoids go untreated, they may prolapse, or protrude, through the anus. This can happen during a bowel movement, or when lifting something heavy. Prolapsed hemorrhoids can be very painful. They may bleed, and can be difficult to put back in place.

If the hemorrhoids are not put back in place, they may get irritated and inflamed. This can lead to a condition called anal stenosis, or narrowing of the anal opening. Anal stenosis can be painful and make it difficult to have a bowel movement.

Untreated hemorrhoids can also lead to blood clots. This can be painful and can cause bleeding. If the clot is large, it can block the anus. This is called thrombosed hemorrhoids, and can be very painful.

What causes hemorrhoids to flare up?

There are a few things that can cause hemorrhoids to flare up. These can include anything from constipation and diarrhea to pregnancy and obesity. Basically, anything that puts extra pressure on your pelvic floor can cause hemorrhoids to become aggravated.

Constipation is one of the most common causes of hemorrhoids. This is because when you are constipated, you are straining to have a bowel movement. This straining can cause the veins in your anus and rectum to become engorged with blood, which can eventually lead to hemorrhoids.

Diarrhea can also cause hemorrhoids to flare up. This is because when you have diarrhea, your stool is softer and more watery. This can cause you to strain when you are having a bowel movement, which can again lead to the veins in your anus and rectum becoming engorged with blood.

Pregnancy is another common cause of hemorrhoids. This is because during pregnancy, your uterus grows and puts extra pressure on your pelvic floor. This extra pressure can cause the veins in your anus and rectum to become engorged with blood, which can eventually lead to hemorrhoids.

Obesity is another common cause of hemorrhoids. This is because when you are obese, you have more weight on your pelvis. This extra weight can put extra pressure on your pelvic floor, which can again lead to the veins in your anus and rectum becoming engorged with blood.

Basically, anything that puts extra pressure on your pelvic floor can cause hemorrhoids to flare up. This includes things like constipation, diarrhea, pregnancy, and obesity. If you are struggling with hemorrhoids, it is important to talk to your doctor about ways to relieve the pressure on your pelvic floor.

How long is too long for a hemorrhoid to last?

If you're wondering how long is too long for a hemorrhoid to last, the answer unfortunately isn't clear. It depends on the individual, the severity of their hemorrhoids, and a few other factors.

For some people, hemorrhoids may only last a few days before disappearing on their own. Other people may experience chronic hemorrhoids that can last for weeks, months, or even years. And unfortunately, for a small percentage of people, hemorrhoids may become so severe that they require surgery to remove.

There are a few things that can affect how long hemorrhoids last. One is the severity of the hemorrhoids. If they're mild, they may go away on their own after a few days. But if they're more severe, they may take longer to go away or may not go away at all without treatment.

Another factor is the individual's lifestyle. People who consume a lot of processed foods and don't get enough fiber or water are more likely to get hemorrhoids. That's because these things can make it difficult for stool to pass through the intestines, which can put extra pressure on the veins in the anus and rectum.

Finally, your hemorrhoids may last longer if you have a history of constipation or other gastrointestinal problems. That's because these conditions can also cause extra pressure on the veins in the anus and rectum.

If you're concerned about how long your hemorrhoids are lasting, talk to your doctor. They can examine your hemorrhoids and give you a better idea of what to expect. In some cases, they may recommend treatment to help speed up the healing process.

There are many possible causes of hemorrhoids, but the most common is straining during bowel movements. Hemorrhoids can be painful, itchy, and can sometimes bleed. Luckily, there are many effective treatments available. In most cases, hemorrhoids can be treated at home with over-the-counter creams and ointments. In more severe cases, surgery may be necessary.

What foods trigger hemorrhoids?

Hemorrhoids are swollen and inflamed blood vessels in the anus and rectum. They can be caused by straining during bowel movements, sitting for long periods of time, or pregnancy. Hemorrhoids can be very painful, and can sometimes bleed.

There are a number of different foods that can trigger hemorrhoids. Eating a high-fiber diet can help to prevent hemorrhoids, but sometimes even foods that are high in fiber can cause them. Foods that can trigger hemorrhoids include:

-Spicy food

-High-fat food

-Acidic food

-Coffee

-Alcohol

Spicy food can trigger hemorrhoids because it can cause irritation and inflammation in the intestine. High-fat food can trigger hemorrhoids because it can lead to constipation, which can then cause hemorrhoids. Acidic food can trigger hemorrhoids because it can irritate the lining of the intestine. Coffee can trigger hemorrhoids because it can lead to dehydration, which can then cause hemorrhoids. Alcohol can trigger hemorrhoids because it can lead to dehydration, which can then cause hemorrhoids.

What's the difference between hemorrhoids and polyps?

There are a few key differences between hemorrhoids and polyps. For one, hemorrhoids are usually located externally, while polyps are located internally. Hemorrhoids are also usually swollen and/or inflamed, while polyps are not. Finally, hemorrhoids can often be painful, while polyps are typically not.

In terms of similarities, both hemorrhoids and polyps can bleed. They can also both cause problems with bowel movements, such as pain and/or bleeding.

What does a hemorrhoid look like?

A hemorrhoid is an enlarged, bulging blood vessel in the anal or rectal area. These vessels can become enlarged and bulging from increased pressure, such as from straining during a bowel movement. Hemorrhoids may be painful, itchy, and can sometimes bleed.")

Hemorrhoids are typically swollen and irritated blood vessels located in the anal or rectal region. They can range in size from small, swollen veins to large, bulging lumps. Many people experience hemorrhoids at some point in their lives, but they usually go away on their own after a few days.

There are a number of things that can cause hemorrhoids, including straining during a bowel movement, sitting for long periods of time, and pregnancy. Hemorrhoids may be painful, itchy, and can sometimes bleed. If you experience any of these symptoms, you should see your doctor to rule out other possible causes and to get treatment.

Treatment for hemorrhoids typically involves a combination of home remedies and over-the-counter (OTC) creams or ointments. In some cases, surgery may be necessary. Home remedies for hemorrhoids include taking a sitz bath, using Witch Hazel pads, and eating more fiber. OTC treatments include creams, ointments, and suppositories that are applied to the affected area. If home remedies and OTC treatments don't work, your doctor may recommend a hemorrhoidectomy, which is surgery to remove the hemorrhoids.

How do you get rid of hemorrhoids in 48 hours?

There are a few things you can do to get rid of hemorrhoids in 48 hours. First, try to avoid constipation by eating a high-fiber diet and drinking plenty of fluids. This will help reduce the pressure on your hemorrhoids. Second, you can try over-the-counter hemorrhoid creams or ointments to help relieve the pain and swelling. Lastly, your doctor may recommend a short course of steroids to help reduce the inflammation.

Can you push hemorrhoids back in?

Hemorrhoids are a sensitive topic for many people. It can be quite embarrassing to talk about them with anyone, even a doctor. So, can you push hemorrhoids back in?

The answer is yes and no. If your hemorrhoids are merely prolapsed, meaning they have fallen out of the rectum but are still attached, then yes, you can push them back in. However, if your hemorrhoids are thrombosed, meaning they have a blood clot, you should not attempt to push them back in. This could cause the clot to break free and cause more bleeding.

If your hemorrhoids are prolapsed, there are a few things you can do to try and reduce the swelling and keep them from falling out again. You can try sitting in a warm sitz bath for 15-20 minutes several times a day. You can also apply a hemorrhoidal cream or ointment to the area. These can soothe the area and provide some relief from the discomfort.

If your hemorrhoids are thrombosed, you will likely need to see a doctor to have them treated. There are a few things that can be done to ease the pain and discomfort in the meantime. You can take a sitz bath as usual, but you may also need to take over the counter pain medication. You should also avoid sitting for long periods of time, as this can exacerbate the pain.

If you are struggling with hemorrhoids, know that you are not alone. Many people suffer from this condition and there are ways to find relief. Talk to your doctor about the best course of treatment for your individual situation.

Can a hemorrhoid burst?

A hemorrhoid is an enlarged vein in the lower rectum and/or anus. When they are inflamed, they can itch, bleed, and be very painful. In some cases, the individual may feel as if they have a bowel movement, but no stool is passed.

There are two types of hemorrhoids: internal and external. Internal hemorrhoids are located inside the rectum. They usually do not hurt, but they can bleed. External hemorrhoids are located under the skin around the anus. They usually are painful and may bleed.

A hemorrhoid may burst if it is scratched, rubbed, or pulled too hard. This can cause bleeding and pain. If a hemorrhoid bursts, it can be very dangerous. You should see a doctor as soon as possible if this happens.

Can hemorrhoids be cancerous?

Hemorrhoids can be cancerous, but it is not a common occurrence. If you have hemorrhoids, you may be at a higher risk for developing anal cancer, but the risk is still relatively low. According to the American Cancer Society, the lifetime risk of developing anal cancer is about 1 in 500 for women and 1 in 200 for men. However, the vast majority of hemorrhoids are not cancerous.

There are a few things that can increase your risk of developing anal cancer, such as HPV (human papillomavirus) infection, smoking, and immunosuppression. HPV is a very common virus that is spread through sexual contact. There are many different types of HPV, and some of them can cause cancer. If you have anal sex, you are at a higher risk for HPV infection, and if you have multiple partners, your risk goes up even more. Smoking cigarettes can also increase your risk of anal cancer. The chemicals in cigarettes can damage the DNA in cells, which can lead to cancer. Immunosuppression (a weakened immune system) can also increase your risk of developing anal cancer. This can be caused by things like HIV infection, organ transplantation, and certain types of chemotherapy.

If you have any risk factors for anal cancer, it's important to talk to your doctor. They may recommend that you have regular anal cancer screenings, which can help catch the disease early. The earlier anal cancer is caught, the easier it is to treat.

In conclusion, hemorrhoids are a common condition that can be very painful. They can be caused by constipation, pregnancy, or straining during bowel movements. Hemorrhoids can be treated with over-the-counter creams, suppositories, or ointments. In severe cases, surgery may be necessary.

What size hemorrhoids need surgery?

Most people with hemorrhoids don't need surgery. However, you may need surgery if your hemorrhoids are very large and painful or if you have bleeding. Surgery can be done in several ways, depending on your situation and the severity of your hemorrhoids.

If you have hemorrhoids, surgery may be an option if:

-Your hemorrhoids are very large.

-You have surgery to remove hemorrhoids that keep returning.

-You have both internal and external hemorrhoids.

-You have bleeding from your hemorrhoids.

-Your hemorrhoids are causing pain or making it difficult to go to the bathroom.

-You have other medical conditions that make hemorrhoid surgery more risky.

Hemorrhoid surgery is usually done on an outpatient basis, which means you can go home the same day. The type of surgery you have will depend on the severity of your hemorrhoids.

You may need a hemorrhoidectomy to remove hemorrhoids. This is a procedure to remove hemorrhoids that are located inside the rectum.

You may need a hemorrhoidectomy to remove hemorrhoids that are located outside the rectum.

You may need a hemorrhoidectomy to remove both internal and external hemorrhoids.

How long does it take for a hemorrhoid to shrink?

A hemorrhoid is an swollen blood vessel in the lower rectum or anus. Despite their name, they are not caused by excess booze. They can, however, be brought on by pregnancy, diarrhea, and constipation—as well as sitting on the toilet for long periods of time, according to the Mayo Clinic.

When these blood vessels become dilated, they can form a lump on the anus, which can be painful. If you've ever had one, you know they're not pleasant. But how long do they last?

"Most hemorrhoids will improve with home treatment in a week or two," notes the Mayo Clinic. So, if you're dealing with a hemorrhoid, you can expect it to take about two weeks for it to shrink.

There are a few home treatments you can try to speed up the process. The Mayo Clinic suggests:

- soaking your bottom in a tub of warm water for 10 to 15 minutes a few times a day

- applying a hemorrhoid cream or ointment to the affected area

- using over-the-counter wipes or pads that are soaked in witch hazel or a similar soothing agent

- placing a small, doughnut-shaped cushion on your bottom when you sit

If your hemorrhoids don't go away after a couple of weeks, or if they cause pain and bleeding, you may need to see a doctor. They can prescribe medication or, in some cases, perform minor surgery to remove the hemorrhoids.

But in most cases, hemorrhoids will go away on their own within a few weeks. So, if you're dealing with one, hang in there—relief is on the way.

Can stress cause hemorrhoids?

Stress is not generally considered a cause of hemorrhoids, but it can aggravate the condition. If you already have hemorrhoids, stress can make them worse. Symptoms of hemorrhoids can include itching, burning, pain, and bleeding. hemorrhoids are caused by increased pressure in the anal or rectal veins. This pressure can be from pregnancy, obesity, straining during bowel movements, or sitting for long periods of time.

Stress does not typically cause hemorrhoids, but it can make the condition worse. If you have hemorrhoids, stress can worsen your symptoms. Hemorrhoid symptoms can include itching, burning, pain, and bleeding.

Hemorrhoids are caused by increased pressure in the anal or rectal veins. This pressure can come from pregnancy, obesity, straining during bowel movements, or sitting for long periods of time.

If you have hemorrhoids and are experiencing stress, there are a few things you can do to ease your symptoms. You can try over-the-counter hemorrhoid creams or ointments, take a sitz bath, or use moistened toilet paper. If your symptoms are severe, you may need to see a doctor for treatment.

Should I go to the doctor with hemorrhoids?

There is no sure answer to this question. Some people with hemorrhoids never experience any symptoms, while others may experience mild symptoms that do not require treatment from a doctor. However, if you experience severe symptoms such as bleeding from the anus, rectal pain, or a prolapsed hemorrhoid (a hemorrhoid that protrudes from the anus), then you should see a doctor. These symptoms may indicate a more serious condition, such as an anal fissure, and a doctor will be able to properly diagnose and treat you.

Does walking make hemorrhoids worse?

Hemorrhoids are swollen blood vessels in the lower rectum or anus. They can be uncomfortable and sometimes painful. Walking can make hemorrhoids worse by increasing the pressure on them. This can cause them to bleed or prolapse, which is when they bulge out of the anus. If you have hemorrhoids, you may want to avoid walking or take breaks often to reduce the pressure on them. You should also talk to your doctor about ways to treat your hemorrhoids.

Why won't my external hemorrhoid go away?

External hemorrhoids are not easy to get rid of and often require multiple treatments. There are a number of reasons why your external hemorrhoid may not be going away.

Firstly, it is important to note that external hemorrhoids are usually larger and more painful than internal hemorrhoids. This is because the external hemorrhoids are located outside of the anal sphincter and are therefore more likely to be aggravated and irritated.

There are a number of over-the-counter treatments that can be effective in reducing the inflammation and pain associated with external hemorrhoids.

However, these treatments will not necessarily get rid of the hemorrhoid completely.

If you are still experiencing pain and inflammation after trying over-the-counter treatments, you may need to see a doctor or other medical professional. They will be able to prescribe stronger medication, which may be necessary to get rid of the hemorrhoid completely.

In some cases, surgery may be required to remove the external hemorrhoid. This is usually only necessary if the hemorrhoid is very large or is causing severe pain and discomfort.

If you are struggling to get rid of an external hemorrhoid, it is important to seek medical advice. There are a number of effective treatments available, but it may take some time to find the one that is right for you.

What is the best prescription medicine for hemorrhoids?

There are several prescription medicines that can be effective in treating hemorrhoids. In general, these medicines can be divided into two main categories: those that work to reduce inflammation and those that work to reduce the size of the hemorrhoids.

Some of the most common prescription medicines that are used to treat hemorrhoids include corticosteroids, which are anti-inflammatory medications, and#8232; bulk-forming laxatives, which help to reduce the size of the hemorrhoids. Other common prescription medicines include rubber band ligation, which works to cut off the blood supply to the hemorrhoids, and#8232; and surgery, which is used in more severe cases.

The best prescription medicine for hemorrhoids will vary depending on the individual. However, in general, the medicines that work to reduce inflammation are typically the most effective. This is because inflammation is often the main cause of the pain and discomfort associated with hemorrhoids.

If you are suffering from hemorrhoids, it is important to talk to your doctor to find out which prescription medicine is right for you.

If you have hemorrhoids, you are not alone. Hemorrhoids are a common condition that can be very painful and uncomfortable. However, there are many treatments available that can help. Talk to your doctor about your options and find the best treatment for you.

How do I know if I have piles?

There are a few common symptoms associated with piles, or hemorrhoids. These include bleeding during or after bowel movements, itching or irritation in the anal area, and lumps or masses around the anus.

In some cases, piles can also cause pain or discomfort, especially if they are large and / or prolapsed. This can make it difficult or even painful to sit down, and can also interfere with daily activities such as walking or passing stool.

If you are experiencing any of these symptoms, it is important to see your doctor for a proper diagnosis. They will be able to determine whether you have piles, and if so, what treatment options are available to you.

Are piles serious?

Many people worry about whether piles are serious, but the condition is actually quite common and usually not severe. Hemorrhoids, or hemorrhoids, are swollen blood vessels in the anal canal. They can be painful and uncomfortable, but they are usually not dangerous.

There are two types of hemorrhoids: internal and external. Internal hemorrhoids are located inside the rectum and usually do not cause pain. External hemorrhoids are located under the skin around the anus and can often be painful.

Hemorrhoids are usually caused by increased pressure in the anal canal, which can be due to constipation, pregnancy, childbirth, obesity, or straining during bowel movements. Sometimes, hemorrhoids can be caused by anal fissures, which are small tears in the anal canal.

Hemorrhoids are typically treated with lifestyle changes, such as eating a high-fiber diet, drinking plenty of fluids, and exercise. If these measures do not improve the symptoms of hemorrhoids, there are several medical treatments that can be effective, such as:

-Stool softeners to reduce constipation

-Topical creams or ointments to reduce pain and inflammation

-Sitz baths to soothe the area

-Laser or infrared coagulation to shrink the hemorrhoids

-Rubber band ligation to cut off the blood supply to the hemorrhoids

-Hemorrhoidectomy, a surgery to remove the hemorrhoids

Most people with hemorrhoids do not need surgery, and the condition usually improves with lifestyle changes and medical treatment. However, if hemorrhoids are very large, painful, or bleeding, you should see a doctor to make sure there are no other underlying medical conditions.

How long do piles take to heal?

Piles, or hemorrhoids, are swelling and inflammation of the veins in the anal and rectal areas. They can be extremely painful and can make everyday activities, such as sitting or going to the bathroom, very difficult. Piles are often caused by straining during a bowel movement or from sitting on the toilet for too long. Thankfully, there are a number of things you can do to ease the discomfort and speed up the healing process.

1. Take a sitz bath.

A sitz bath is a warm, shallow bath that can help to soothe the pain and inflammation of piles. You can do this by filling a tub with a few inches of warm water and sitting in it for 10-15 minutes. You can also add Epsom salt, which can help to reduce swelling.

2. Apply a cold compress.

Applying a cold compress to the affected area can also help to reduce pain and swelling. Simply wrap a cold pack or a bag of frozen peas in a towel and apply it to the area for 10-15 minutes.

3. Use over-the-counter creams and ointments.

There are a number of over-the-counter creams and ointments that can help to ease the symptoms of piles. Look for products that contain Witch Hazel or a similar ingredient. Apply the cream or ointment to the affected area several times a day.

4. Try stool softeners.

If constipation is a contributing factor to your piles, then stool softeners can be helpful. These products work by making it easier to pass stools, which can help to reduce straining.

5. Eat plenty of fiber.

A high-fiber diet can also help to reduce constipation and prevent straining. Fiber can be found in fruits, vegetables, and whole grains. You should aim to consume 25-30 grams of fiber per day.

6. Drink plenty of fluids.

Drinking plenty of fluids, especially water, is important for preventing constipation. Aim to drink eight glasses of water per day.

7. Avoid sitting for long periods of time.

If you have to sit for long periods of time, such as at a desk or in a car, try to get up and move around every 30 minutes or so. This will help to keep your blood flowing and prevent pooling of blood in the veins.

8. Try over-the-counter pain relievers.

If the pain of piles is severe, you can try over-the-counter pain relievers, such as ibuprofen or acetaminophen.

9. See your doctor.

If home treatment doesn't seem to be helping

What piles look like?

Piles, or hemorrhoids, are lumps that protrude from the anus. They can be either internal or external and often cause bleeding during bowel movements. They can be very painful and cause a great deal of discomfort.

Piles vary in size and can be as small as a pea or as large as a grape. They can be flesh-colored or purple and often protrude from the anus. External piles can be very painful and cause itchiness and bleeding. Internal piles are often less painful but can still cause bleeding.

Piles are caused by a variety of things, including pregnancy, obesity, constipation, and straining during bowel movements. Treatment for piles depends on the severity of the symptoms and can range from over-the-counter creams to surgery.

Can piles clear up on their own?

It's a common question: can hemorrhoids clear up on their own? The answer is yes, but sometimes they don't.

Hemorrhoids, also known as piles, are swollen veins in the anal canal. They happen when the blood vessels around your anus or rectum become dilated or enlarged. This can happen for a number of reasons, including pregnancy, straining during a bowel movement, or sitting for long periods of time.

The symptoms of hemorrhoids vary, but can include itching, burning, and bleeding. If you have bleeding hemorrhoids, you may notice blood in your stool or on the toilet paper after a bowel movement.

Hemorrhoids are usually not painful, but they can be uncomfortable. Fortunately, there are a number of things you can do to ease the symptoms. These include:

- soaking in a warm bath

- applying a hemorrhoid cream or ointment

- taking over-the-counter pain relievers

If your symptoms are severe, you may need to see a doctor. There are a number of treatment options available, including:

- rubber band ligation, which involves tying a rubber band around the base of the hemorrhoid to cut off its blood supply

- injections, which can help reduce inflammation

- infrared coagulation, which uses heat to destroy the hemorrhoid

- surgery, in severe cases

Most people with hemorrhoids will not need surgery. In most cases, the symptoms will go away on their own with home treatment. However, if your symptoms are severe or persistent, you should see a doctor for treatment.

Can you push piles back in?

Hemorrhoids are a common condition that can cause a lot of discomfort. They are basically swollen blood vessels in the anal area that can bleed and be very painful. Sometimes, people can be unsure about whether or not they should try to push their hemorrhoids back in. Here is some information that may help you make a decision.

The short answer to the question is: generally, no, you should not try to push your hemorrhoids back in. This is because doing so can actually make them worse and more painful. Hemorrhoids are already quite sensitive, so pushing them back in can cause them to bleed and become even more inflamed.

There are a few exceptions to this rule. If your hemorrhoids are only slightly prolapsed, meaning that they have only popped out a little bit, then it is usually okay to gently push them back in. However, you should only do this if it is not painful and you are very careful.

If your hemorrhoids are more severely prolapsed, or if they are causing you a lot of pain, then it is best to leave them alone and see a doctor. A doctor can help you determine the best course of treatment, which may involve a hemorrhoidectomy (surgery to remove the hemorrhoids).

In conclusion, unless your hemorrhoids are only slightly prolapsed, it is generally best to leave them alone and consult a doctor. Pushing them back in can cause them to bleed and become more inflamed, which will only make the situation worse.

Can piles heal on its own?

Hemorrhoids are a common and uncomfortable condition that can develop when the blood vessels in and around your anus become swollen and inflamed. Although hemorrhoids often clear up on their own, they can also be a recurring problem.

There are a number of things you can do to relieve the symptoms of hemorrhoids and help them to heal. These include:

-Avoiding straining when you go to the toilet

-Eating a high-fiber diet

-Drinking plenty of fluids

-Doing regular exercise

-Taking over-the-counter pain relievers

-Applying hemorrhoid cream or ointment

In some cases, hemorrhoids may require more extensive treatment. If your hemorrhoids are large and painful, your doctor may recommend that you have them surgically removed. This is known as hemorrhoidectomy.

If you have hemorrhoids, it is important to see your doctor so that they can rule out other potential causes of your symptoms.

What happens if you don't treat piles?

If left untreated, hemorrhoids can worsen. The tissue around the hemorrhoid can become inflamed and irritated, and the hemorrhoid may become thrombosed, meaning that the blood supply to the hemorrhoid is cut off. This can cause severe pain and may require surgical intervention. Further, if the tissue around the hemorrhoid is repeatedly irritated, it can lead to anal fissures, which are small tears in the tissue. Anal fissures can be extremely painful and may require medical treatment. In extreme cases, untreated hemorrhoids can lead to rectal prolapse, in which the rectum itself prolapses through the anus. This is a very serious condition that can require surgery to correct.

Do piles stay permanently?

It is a common misconception that hemorrhoids always stay permanently. However, in reality, this is not the case. While hemorrhoids may often become permanently prolapsed, or stick out, from the anal opening, they can be pushed back inside. Prolapsed hemorrhoids that cannot be pushed back inside are often removed with surgery.

Should I ignore piles?

Ignoring piles, or hemorrhoids, can have disastrous consequences. Piles are generally the result of straining during bowel movements, pregnancy, or obesity. The increased pressure on the veins in the anal region causes them to bulge and swell. In some cases, blood clots can form. When these blood clots become thrombosed, they can be very painful. If left untreated, piles can lead to serious bleeding, infection, and even anal fistulas.

There are a number of effective treatments for piles, including over-the-counter creams and ointments, stool softeners, and sitz baths. If these conservative measures don't work, your doctor may recommend a more aggressive approach, such as rubber band ligation, sclerotherapy, or hemorrhoidectomy.

Don't suffer in silence if you think you may have piles. Make an appointment to see your doctor. With proper treatment, piles can be managed and may even go away on their own.

How

do I

fix piles fast?

Around 50% of the adult population will suffer from hemorrhoids at some point in their lives. hemorrhoids are veins in the anus and rectum that become swollen and inflamed. They can be either internal or external. Internal hemorrhoids are usually painless but can cause bleeding during bowel movements. External hemorrhoids can be very painful.

There are a number of things you can do to ease the symptoms of hemorrhoids. Taking a warm bath can help to reduce pain and inflammation. Over-the-counter creams and ointments can also be effective. If your hemorrhoids are severe, you may need to see a doctor for treatment. Surgery is sometimes necessary to remove hemorrhoids.

What cream gets rid of piles?

There are a number of different creams that can be effective in getting rid of piles, though which one will work best for you may depend on the severity of your condition. For milder cases, a over-the-counter cream may be enough to provide relief, while more severe cases may require a prescription-strength cream.

One of the most popular over-the-counter creams for piles is Preparation H. This cream contains ingredients that help to soothe and protect the skin, reduce inflammation, and shrink the size of hemorrhoids. It is available in a variety of forms, including regular ointment, ointment with an applicator, medicated wipes, and suppositories.

Another popular choice is Anusol, which contains similar active ingredients to Preparation H. This cream is available in both ointment and suppository form. It can be used to relieve pain, itching, and swelling associated with hemorrhoids, and can also help to shrink the size of hemorrhoids.

For more severe cases of hemorrhoids, a prescription-strength cream may be necessary. These creams typically contain a higher concentration of active ingredients than over-the-counter options, and can be more effective in reducing inflammation and shrinking hemorrhoids.

If you are suffering from hemorrhoids, speak to your doctor or pharmacist about which cream may be best for you.

What's the best medication for piles?

There are several different medications that can be used to treat piles, and the best one for you will depend on your individual circumstances. If you have mild piles, you may be able to treat them with over-the-counter medications like creams or ointments. If your piles are more severe, you may need to see a doctor for prescription medication.

There are a few different types of medication that can be used to treat piles. cream or ointment, for example, can be applied directly to the affected area to soothe discomfort and reduce swelling. If your piles are internal, you may be prescribed a suppository, which is a small capsule that is inserted into the rectum. Some oral medications can also be used to treat piles, although these are not typically the first choice.

The best medication for piles will depend on the severity of your condition. For mild piles, over-the-counter treatments may be all that you need. If your piles are more severe, your doctor may prescribe a stronger medication. In some cases, surgery may be the best option.

Do piles get bigger?

Hemorrhoids are often described as varicose veins in the anus or rectum. They can be internal, which means they are inside the rectum. Or they can be external, which means they are outside of the anus. Hemorrhoids are usually the result of straining during a bowel movement, pregnancy, or from being overweight.

It's common for hemorrhoids to enlarge, bleed, and itch. In some cases, they can even become thrombosed, or filled with blood clots. If this happens, it can be extremely painful. If you have any of these symptoms, you should see a doctor right away.

There are a few things that you can do to try to prevent hemorrhoids from occurring in the first place. For one, you can take steps to avoid constipation. This means eating a high-fiber diet, drinking plenty of fluids, and exercising regularly. You should also avoid sitting or standing for long periods of time. If you are pregnant, you can try to prevent hemorrhoids by not straining during bowel movements and by not sitting for long periods of time.

If you already have hemorrhoids, there are a few things that you can do to ease the symptoms. You can soak the area in warm water for 10-15 minutes several times a day. This can help to soothe the pain and itching. You can also use over-the-counter creams or ointments to help relieve the symptoms. If these things don't work, or if your symptoms are severe, you may need to see a doctor. A doctor can prescribe stronger medications, or even surgery, to help get rid of the hemorrhoids.

Hemorrhoids are a common and painful affliction that can be treated effectively at home with over the counter remedies or by seeking medical attention. Left untreated, they can cause serious health complications. While they are often embarrassing to talk about, hemorrhoids are nothing to be ashamed of and are a very common condition.

Can you live with untreated hemorrhoids?

Hemorrhoids are a very common condition that millions of people suffer from. While they may be painful and cause a lot of discomfort, they are not usually a serious condition. In most cases, they can be treated at home with over-the-counter medications or home remedies. However, in some cases, hemorrhoids can become so severe that they require medical treatment.

If you have hemorrhoids, you may be wondering if you can live with them untreated. The truth is, it is possible to live with untreated hemorrhoids, but it is not recommended. Untreated hemorrhoids can become very painful and lead to bleeding. They can also cause anal fissures, which are small tears in the anal canal. These fissures can be very painful and can make it difficult to have a bowel movement. In some cases, untreated hemorrhoids can also lead to blood clots. If a blood clot forms in an external hemorrhoid, it can be very painful and may require medical treatment.

If you have hemorrhoids, it is important to talk to your doctor about treatment options. There are many different treatments available, and your doctor can help you choose the best option for you.

What is the last stage of hemorrhoids?

The last stage of hemorrhoids is marked by a prolapse, or the \emph{slip-ping}

of hemorrhoids from the rectum. This can cause bleeding, pain, and

irritation. Prolapsed hemorrhoids may go back inside on their own, or

may need to be pushed back in. If prolapsed hemorrhoids cannot be pushed

back in, surgery may be necessary.

What not to drink when you have hemorrhoids?

There are a few things to keep in mind when it comes to what not to drink when you have hemorrhoids. For one, caffeine can act as a diuretic and lead to dehydration. This is the last thing you want when you're suffering from hemorrhoids, as dehydration can make your condition worse.

Alcohol is also a diuretic, so it's best to avoid drinking it if you have hemorrhoids. In addition, drinking alcohol can also lead to dehydration, which as we mentioned, is something you want to avoid if you have hemorrhoids.

It's also important to avoid drinking anything that's too hot or too cold. Extreme temperatures can aggravate hemorrhoids, so it's best to stick to lukewarm beverages.

All in all, when it comes to what not to drink when you have hemorrhoids, it's best to steer clear of caffeine, alcohol, and extreme temperatures. Stick to drinking plenty of water and other lukewarm fluids to keep your body hydrated and avoid aggravating your hemorrhoids.

What food shrinks hemorrhoids fast?

There are a few different things that you can do in order to shrink hemorrhoids quickly. For one, you can increase your fiber intake by eating more fiber-rich foods or taking a fiber supplement. This will help to soften your stools and make them easier to pass, which can reduce the amount of irritation to your hemorrhoids. You can also try sitting in a warm bath for 10-15 minutes to help reduce the swelling.

Another thing that can help to shrink hemorrhoids quickly is to apply a cold compress to the area for a few minutes several times a day. This can help to numb the area and reduce the inflammation. If you have hemorrhoids that are particularly large or painful, your doctor may also recommend a procedure called ligation, which involves tying off the blood vessels to the hemorrhoids to reduce blood flow to the area and shrink the hemorrhoids.

What exercises help hemorrhoids?

Hemorrhoids are one of the most common Anal Fissure problems. They are caused by strained bowel movements, sitting for long periods of time on the toilet, or pregnancy. Hemorrhoids can be very painful, and sometimes bleed.

There are a few different exercises that can help relieve the pain and discomfort of hemorrhoids. These exercises can also help to prevent hemorrhoids from developing in the first place.

One simple exercise that can help with hemorrhoids is to sit on a hard surface and raise your legs up in the air. This helps to increase the blood flow to the area and can reduce the swelling.

Another exercise that can help is to lie on your back and bring your knees up to your chest. This helps to take the pressure off of the area and can also help to increase blood flow.

If you are pregnant, there are special exercises that can help to relieve the pressure on the area. One of these is to lie on your back and put a pillow under your knees. This helps to take the pressure off of your pelvis and can also help with hemorrhoids.

There are also a few dietary changes that can help with hemorrhoids.eating high-fiber foods, drinking plenty of water, and avoiding constipation.

Do you need a colonoscopy for hemorrhoids?

A colonoscopy is a medical procedure that allows your doctor to examine the lining of your large intestine (colon) for abnormal growths, polyps, or other abnormalities. A colonoscopy can also be used to diagnose and treat certain intestinal conditions, such as hemorrhoids.

While most colonoscopies are performed for preventive screening or to investigate potential cancer concerns, you may need a colonoscopy to diagnose and treat hemorrhoids. Hemorrhoids are swollen blood vessels in the lower rectum and anus. They can be painful and bleed during bowel movements.

If your doctor suspects that you have hemorrhoids, they will likely recommend a colonoscopy to confirm the diagnosis. During a colonoscopy, your doctor will insert a flexible, lighted tube into your rectum and colon. The tube has a camera attached to it, which allows your doctor to get a close-up view of the inside of your colon.

Your doctor may also take biopsies during a colonoscopy. Biopsies are small samples of tissue that are removed during the procedure and then examined under a microscope. This can help your doctor to rule out other conditions, such as colorectal cancer.

After your colonoscopy, you will likely be able to go home the same day. You may experience some cramping and bloating as the air that was used to inflate your colon during the procedure is passed out of your body. You should be able to return to your normal activities the next day.

If your colonoscopy does confirm that you have hemorrhoids, your doctor will likely recommend treatment to relieve your symptoms. Treatment options for hemorrhoids include dietary changes, over-the-counter medications, and/or surgery. Surgery is typically only recommended for severe cases of hemorrhoids that do not respond to other treatment methods.

If you have hemorrhoids, you may be wondering if you need a colonoscopy. While a colonoscopy is not always necessary, it may be recommended by your doctor to confirm the diagnosis and/or to rule out other conditions. If your doctor suspects that you have hemorrhoids, they will likely recommend a colonoscopy to confirm the diagnosis. During a colonoscopy, your doctor will insert a flexible, lighted tube into your rectum and colon. The tube has a camera attached to it, which allows your doctor to get a close-up view of the inside of your colon. Your doctor may also take biopsies during a colonoscopy. Biopsies are small samples of tissue that are removed during the procedure and then examined under a microscope. This can help your doctor to rule out other conditions, such as colorectal cancer.

What is the main cause of piles?

Most cases of hemorrhoids are caused by straining during bowel movements. This happens when the muscles in your pelvic floor contract to prop up your intestines and hold in stool. When those muscles are strained, blood vessels in your anus and rectum can become swollen and bulge. This can cause bleeding, pain, and irritation.

Other causes of hemorrhoids include pregnancy, aging, chronic constipation or diarrhea, and anal intercourse. Anything that puts extra pressure on your anal or rectal area can cause hemorrhoids. This includes sitting on the toilet for a long time, standing or lifting objects, and straining to have a bowel movement.

If you have any of these risk factors, you may be more likely to develop hemorrhoids. That doesn't mean you'll definitely get them, but it's important to be aware of the potential.

Hemorrhoids are a painful and annoying problem that afflict many people. Although there are many treatments available, the best way to avoid hemorrhoids is to prevent them in the first place. To do this, eat a high-fiber diet, drink plenty of water, and exercise regularly.

What cream shrinks external hemorrhoids?

There are a few different creams that can be used to help shrink external hemorrhoids. One option is to use a hemorrhoid cream that contains corticosteroids. This can help to reduce the inflammation and swelling associated with the hemorrhoids. Another option is to use a cream that contains video dock, which is a natural plant extract that has been shown to be effective in reducing the size of hemorrhoids.

Can ibuprofen help shrink hemorrhoids?

Yes, ibuprofen can help reduce the size of hemorrhoids. Ibuprofen is an anti-inflammatory medication, so it can help to reduce the swelling around the hemorrhoids. This can help to make the hemorrhoids smaller and less uncomfortable.

If you are thinking about taking ibuprofen to help with your hemorrhoids, it is important to speak to a doctor first. This is because ibuprofen can interact with other medications, and it may not be suitable for everyone.

In general, ibuprofen is a safe and effective medication for reducing the size of hemorrhoids. However, it is always important to speak to a doctor before taking any medication, to make sure it is safe for you and will not interact with any other medication you are taking.

Does squeezing a hemorrhoid help?

Hemorrhoids are often uncomfortable and can be quite painful. Sometimes, people with hemorrhoids may try to find relief by squeezing the affected area. But does this actually help?

There is no one definitive answer to this question. In some cases, squeezing a hemorrhoid may provide temporary relief from pain and/or itchiness. However, it is important to remember that hemorrhoids are often irritated by excessive rubbing and squeezing, so this relief may only be temporary.

In other cases, squeezing a hemorrhoid may actually make the symptoms worse. This is because hemorrhoids are often already quite sensitive, and squeezing them can further irritate the area. If the hemorrhoid is particularly large or painful, squeezing it may also cause it to rupture. This can lead to even more pain and discomfort.

If you are considering squeezing a hemorrhoid, it is important to talk to your doctor first. They can help you determine whether or not this is likely to be a helpful or harmful treatment for your individual case.

How many hours is hemorrhoid surgery?

Surgery to remove hemorrhoids is called a hemorrhoidectomy. The surgery takes about 1 to 2 hours. You will be given a general anesthetic to keep you asleep during the surgery.

During the surgery, the doctor removes the tissue around the hemorrhoids. This may be done with a scalpel, a laser, or a cautery instrument. The tissue is then stitched closed. A hemorrhoidectomy is usually done as an outpatient procedure. This means you can go home the same day.

If you have large hemorrhoids, you may need to stay in the hospital for 1 or 2 days. You may have some bleeding from your rectum for the first week or so after surgery. Your doctor will probably tell you to take a stool softener to make it easier. You may also have some pain and need to take pain medication for a week or two.

It is normal to have some sores around your anus for a few weeks after surgery. These usually heal on their own. The surgery site may also be sore for a while. You may need to take a short course of antibiotics to prevent infection.

What is a Stage 3 hemorrhoid?

A hemorrhoid is a stage 3 when it prolapses and becomes evident outside the anal canal. At this stage, the hemorrhoid cannot be pushed back inside the anal canal. This is a more serious condition that can cause great discomfort. If you have a stage 3 hemorrhoid, it is important to see a doctor right away so that you can get the proper treatment.

How long do you stay in hospital after hemorrhoid surgery?

After hemorrhoid surgery, you will stay in the hospital for 1-2 days. During this time, you will be monitored closely by the nurses and doctors. You will be given pain medication and will be encouraged to move around as much as possible. Once you are discharged from the hospital, you will need to take it easy for the first few days. Avoid strenuous activity and constipation. Drink plenty of fluids and eat a high-fiber diet.

Can I just leave my hemorrhoids?

Hemorrhoids are a common condition that can cause a lot of discomfort. Many people are wondering if they can just leave their hemorrhoids and not seek treatment. The answer is no, you cannot just leave your hemorrhoids. If you do not seek treatment, the hemorrhoids can get worse and lead to more serious complications.

Hemorrhoids are caused by enlarged veins in the anus and rectum. These veins can become inflamed and cause a lot of discomfort. There are a number of things that can cause hemorrhoids, such as constipation, pregnancy, and obesity. If you have hemorrhoids, you may notice blood in your stool, pain when you poop, and itching around your anus.

There are a number of treatment options for hemorrhoids. If you have mild hemorrhoids, you may be able to treat them at home with over-the-counter creams or suppositories. If you have severe hemorrhoids, you may need to see a doctor for treatment. Treatment options for severe hemorrhoids include rubber band ligation, sclerotherapy, and surgery.

You should not just leave your hemorrhoids untreated. If you do not seek treatment, the hemorrhoids can get worse and lead to more serious complications. If you have hemorrhoids, you should talk to your doctor about the best treatment option for you.

If you have hemorrhoids, you're not alone. Around 75% of Americans will develop hemorrhoids at some point in their lives. Although hemorrhoids can be painful and uncomfortable, they're usually not serious. In most cases, hemorrhoids can be treated with home remedies. If home remedies don't work, you can try medical treatments.

Should you push hemorrhoids in?

Hemorrhoids are lumps of tissue, usually with blood vessels running through them, that form in the anal canal and around the anus. They can be painful, itchy, and bleeding. Sometimes, people with hemorrhoids will try to push them back in, but is that a good idea?

There are a couple of things to consider before trying to push hemorrhoids back in. First, are the hemorrhoids external or internal? External hemorrhoids are those that are right at the anal opening and are usually the most painful. Internal hemorrhoids are inside the anal canal and can be more difficult to deal with. Second, how large are the hemorrhoids? If they are small, it might be possible to push them back in, but if they are large, it might be difficult or even impossible.

If you do decide to try and push your hemorrhoids back in, there are a few things you can do to make it more successful. First, use a lubricant. This will help the hemorrhoids slide back in more easily and decrease the risk of further irritation. Second, try to push them in gently. If you push too hard, you could end up making the hemorrhoids worse. Finally, don't force it. If the hemorrhoids don't want to go back in, don't try to force them. You could end up causing more pain and irritation.

If you're not sure whether or not you should try to push your hemorrhoids back in, it's best to consult with a doctor. They can help you figure out what the best course of action is for your situation.

How long does it take for external hemorrhoids to shrink?

External hemorrhoids are a lot like varicose veins that occur in your legs. They can be uncomfortable and cause itching and bleeding. You may be wondering how long it will take for them to shrink.

It depends on the severity of your hemorrhoids. If they are just enlarged blood vessels, they may go away on their own. But, if they are large and bulging, they may need to be treated.

There are a few things you can do to help shrink hemorrhoids. This includes:

-Eating a high-fiber diet. This will help to bulk up your stool and make it easier to pass. This can also help to prevent constipation, which can worsen hemorrhoids.

-Drinking plenty of fluids. This will help to keep your stool soft and easy to pass.

-Taking over-the-counter medications. These can help to reduce inflammation and pain.

If your hemorrhoids are large and bulging, your doctor may recommend a hemorrhoidectomy. This is a surgery to remove the hemorrhoids. Recovery time from this surgery is usually about two to four weeks.

It is important to talk to your doctor if you are experiencing any rectal bleeding. This could be a sign of a more serious problem.

How do you treat an external hemorrhoid lump?

External hemorrhoids are a common condition that can cause a great deal of discomfort. In most cases, hemorrhoids can be treated at home with over-the-counter creams, ointments, or patches. If the hemorrhoids are particularly large or painful, you may need to see a doctor for a more aggressive treatment.

There are a few different ways to treat an external hemorrhoid lump. The first is to apply a hemorrhoidal cream or ointment to the area. This will help to soothe the pain and inflammation. You can also try using a hemorrhoidal pad or Witch Hazel pad to help reduce swelling. If the lump is very large, you may need to see a doctor for a hemorrhoidectomy, which is a surgical procedure to remove the hemorrhoid.

If you are suffering from an external hemorrhoid lump, there are a few things you can do at home to help ease the pain and discomfort. By following the above tips, you should be able to get rid of the lump and get back to your normal life.

What stage is external hemorrhoids?

There are four stages of external hemorrhoids. The first stage is when the hemorrhoids are swollen and painful, but not too severe. The second stage is when the hemorrhoids are more severe and require more treatment. The third stage is when the hemorrhoids are very severe and require surgery. The fourth stage is when the hemorrhoids are so severe that they need to be removed.

Should I walk with external hemorrhoids?

If you have external hemorrhoids, you may be wondering if you should walk with them. The answer is that it depends. If your hemorrhoids are painful, walking may not be the best activity for you. However, if your hemorrhoids are not painful, walking may help to reduce the size of your hemorrhoids and improve your symptoms.

There are a few things to keep in mind if you decide to walk with your hemorrhoids. First, be sure to wear loose-fitting clothing so that your hemorrhoids are not irritated by tight clothing. Second, avoid walking for long periods of time. If you must walk for long periods of time, take breaks and sit down when you can. Finally, be sure to take it easy when you walk. Do not do any intense exercise or activity that could make your symptoms worse.

Overall, walking is a good activity for most people with hemorrhoids. However, it is important to listen to your body and do what is best for you. If walking is painful, take a break and try another activity.

What happens if you push an external hemorrhoid back in?

If you have an external hemorrhoid, it's likely that at some point you will feel the urge to push it back in. Although this may seem like a harmless act, it can actually cause quite a bit of pain and may even lead to more serious problems.

When you first feel the urge to push your hemorrhoid back in, you will likely experience a sharp pain. This is because the hemorrhoid is being pushed back into the anal canal, where it is not supposed to be. As the hemorrhoid continues to be pushed back, the pain will likely become more intense. In some cases, the act of pushing a hemorrhoid back in can even cause it to rupture. If this happens, you will likely experience even more pain as well as bleeding.

Pushing a hemorrhoid back in can also cause other problems. For instance, if the hemorrhoid is not pushed back in all the way, it may become prolapsed. This means that it will actually protrude from the anal canal. Prolapsed hemorrhoids can be very painful and may require surgery to fix.

So, what happens if you push an external hemorrhoid back in? It's not a good idea. You may experience pain, bleeding, and even more serious problems. It's best to just leave your hemorrhoids alone and let them do their job.

Will an external hemorrhoid go back in on its own?

A hemorrhoid is an enlarged, swollen blood vessel in the anal or rectal area. There are two types of hemorrhoids: internal and external. An internal hemorrhoid is located inside the rectum, while an external hemorrhoid is located under the skin around the anus.

If you have an external hemorrhoid, it is possible that it will go back in on its own. However, this is not always the case, and it is important to see a doctor if your hemorrhoid does not go away or if you experience pain, bleeding, or other symptoms. If you have an internal hemorrhoid, it is not possible for it to go back in on its own, and you should see a doctor if you experience any symptoms.

There are a number of things you can do to treat hemorrhoids and ease your symptoms. These include: taking over-the-counter pain relievers; applying local heat; using stool softeners; and avoiding straining during bowel movements. If these conservative measures don't provide relief, your doctor may suggest other treatments, such as rubber band ligation, sclerotherapy, infrared coagulation, or hemorrhoidectomy.

Can piles burst?

There is a lot of misinformation out there about hemorrhoids, and one of the most common questions is whether or not they can burst. The answer, unfortunately, is a bit complicated.

Hemorrhoids are dilated veins located in the anal canal or rectum, and they can become engorged and enlarged when there is increased pressure in these areas. When this happens, the hemorrhoids can become quite painful. In some cases, the enlarged hemorrhoids can prolapse, or bulge out, through the anal opening.

While hemorrhoids can certainly become quite large, they cannot actually burst in the same way that, say, a balloon can. However, prolapsed hemorrhoids can sometimes become trapped outside of the anal opening, and when this happens, they can bleed quite heavily. If the bleeding is not stopped, hemorrhoids can become quite dry and cracked, and this can lead to pain and even more bleeding.

If you are experiencing any kind of hemorrhoidal bleeding, it is important to see a doctor as soon as possible. In some cases, surgery may be necessary to remove the hemorrhoids. However, in most cases, hemorrhoids can be treated at home with over-the-counter creams, ointments, and pads.

If you are wondering whether or not hemorrhoids can burst, the answer is a bit complicated. In short, they cannot burst in the same way that a balloon can, but they can become trapped outside of the anal opening, which can lead to pain and bleeding. If you are experiencing any kind of hemorrhoidal bleeding, it is important to see a doctor as soon as possible.

When do piles need surgery?

At what point do hemorrhoids become so severe that they require surgery? This is a common question asked by those who suffer from this painful condition.

There are a number of different factors that can contribute to the severity of hemorrhoids. One of the most important factors is the amount of pressure that is being placed on the blood vessels in the anal area. This pressure can be caused by a variety of things, such as constipation, pregnancy, or being overweight.

If the pressure on the blood vessels gets too high, it can cause the vessels to bulge and become enlarged. When this happens, the hemorrhoids can become very painful. They may also bleed, which can cause even more pain.

In most cases, hemorrhoids can be treated with simple home remedies, such as taking over-the-counter pain medication and using stool softeners. These methods can help to relieve the pressure on the blood vessels and reduce the swelling.

However, in some cases, the hemorrhoids may become so severe that these home remedies are not enough to provide relief. When this happens, it may be necessary to see a doctor for more aggressive treatment.

One of the most common options for treating severe hemorrhoids is surgery. This usually involves removing the hemorrhoids entirely. In some cases, the surgeon may also need to remove a small portion of the surrounding tissue.

Surgery is generally considered to be a last resort for treating hemorrhoids. This is because it is a very invasive procedure and can be quite painful. It is also important to note that surgery does not always provide a cure for hemorrhoids. In some cases, the hemorrhoids may return even after surgery.

If you are suffering from severe hemorrhoids, it is important to talk to your doctor about all of your treatment options. Surgery should only be considered if other methods have failed and the hemorrhoids are causing you a great deal of pain.

When should you see a doctor for piles?

There are a few signs that indicate that someone may have piles, and if these signs are present, it is best to see a doctor. These signs include: rectal bleeding, anal pain or itching, lump near the anus, mucus discharge from the anus, or pain during bowel movements. If any of these are present, it is best to see a doctor to get a proper diagnosis, as these symptoms can also be indicative of other conditions.

Piles, also known as hemorrhoids, are when the blood vessels in the anal and rectal area become swollen and inflamed. This can happen for a number of reasons, such as sitting for long periods of time on the toilet, pregnancy, or straining during a bowel movement. Piles can be either internal, meaning they are inside the anal canal, or external, meaning they are outside of the anal canal.

There are a few things that can be done at home to help ease the symptoms of piles, such as taking a warm bath, using a hemorrhoid cream, or avoiding sitting for long periods of time. However, if the symptoms persist, it is best to see a doctor. The doctor will be able to properly diagnose the condition and recommend the best course of treatment. In some cases, surgery may be necessary to remove the hemorrhoids.

Are hemorrhoids cancerous?

Hemorrhoids are unpleasant, but usually not dangerous. They can cause bleeding from the rectum and pain, and sometimes itching, but they will not lead to cancer. In fact, hemorrhoids are often caused by straining during bowel movements, and are more common in people who are constipated. If you have hemorrhoids, you can try over-the-counter creams or ointments to ease the discomfort, and make sure to eat plenty of fiber to keep your stool soft. If the hemorrhoids are persistent or very painful, you may need to see a doctor for treatment.

Do piles get worse with age?

As we age, our bodies go through a lot of changes. Some of these changes can lead to the development of hemorrhoids. But do hemorrhoids necessarily get worse with age?

There are a few things that can contribute to the development of hemorrhoids, such as chronic constipation or diarrhea, obesity, pregnancy, and a sedentary lifestyle. People who have any of these risk factors are more likely to develop hemorrhoids as they age.

There are two types of hemorrhoids: internal and external. Internal hemorrhoids are located inside the rectum and are usually not painful. External hemorrhoids are located under the skin around the anus and can sometimes be painful.

Hemorrhoids are more common in adults over the age of 50, but they can happen at any age. They are more likely to occur in people who have a family history of hemorrhoids.

There are a few things you can do to prevent the development of hemorrhoids, such as eating a high-fiber diet, drinking plenty of fluids, and exercising regularly. If you already have hemorrhoids, there are a few things you can do to ease the symptoms, such as using over-the-counter creams and taking warm baths.

In most cases, hemorrhoids will not get worse with age. However, the risk factors for developing hemorrhoids can increase with age. This is why it's important to take steps to prevent the development of hemorrhoids.

How common is piles?

Hemorrhoids, also known as piles, are a common and painful condition caused by swollen blood vessels in theRectum and anus. The National Institute of Diabetes and Digestive and Kidney Diseases (NIDDK) estimates that 3 million Americans suffer from hemorrhoids each year. Hemorrhoids are more common in adults over the age of 50, but can affect anyone.

There are two types of hemorrhoids: internal and external. Internal hemorrhoids are located inside the anus and are not usually painful. External hemorrhoids are located under the skin around the anus and can be very painful.

Hemorrhoids are common, but not everyone experiences symptoms. The most common symptom of hemorrhoids is bleeding during a bowel movement. Other symptoms include itching, pain, and irritation.

Hemorrhoids are usually not dangerous and can be treated with over-the-counter creams or hemorrhoid cream. If hemorrhoids are severe, surgery may be needed.

There are many treatments for hemorrhoids, including at-home remedies, such as sitz baths and ice packs, as well as over-the-counter creams and ointments. In most cases, hemorrhoids can be treated at home with these simple home remedies. However, occasionally, hemorrhoids may require medical treatment.

What are signs of internal hemorrhoids?

Most people with hemorrhoids experience symptoms at some point. These can include bleeding, anal itching, and pain or discomfort when sitting. Some people also experience prolapse, where the hemorrhoid bulges out of the anus.

Most of the time, hemorrhoids are not painful. However, they can become painful if they prolapse and are pushed back inside, or if a blood clot forms inside them. If this happens, it is called a thrombosed hemorrhoid.

There are several different types of hemorrhoids, depending on where they are located. Internal hemorrhoids are located inside the rectum, while external hemorrhoids are located under the skin around the anus.

There are a few different ways to treat hemorrhoids. One option is to do nothing and wait for them to go away on their own. This often takes a few days to a few weeks.

Another option is to use over-the-counter creams, ointments, or suppositories. These can help to soothe the area and reduce inflammation.

If the hemorrhoids are large and painful, your doctor may recommend a hemorrhoidectomy. This is a surgical procedure to remove the hemorrhoids.

Hemorrhoids are common, and most people will experience them at some point in their lives. while they are usually not painful, they can become painful if they prolapse or a blood clot forms. There are several different treatment options available, so talk to your doctor to find the best one for you.

What shrinks internal hemorrhoid?

There are two main types of hemorrhoids: internal and external. Internal hemorrhoids are located inside the rectum, while external hemorrhoids are located under the skin around the anus.

There are several things that can help shrink internal hemorrhoids. One is to add more fiber to your diet. This can be done by eating more fruits and vegetables, whole grains, and legumes. You should also aim to drink at least eight glasses of water a day. This will help soften your stools and make them easier to pass.

Another way to shrink internal hemorrhoids is to avoid straining during bowel movements. This can be done by making sure you have regular bowel movements, going to the bathroom when you first feel the urge, and avoiding constipation. You can also try to use a stool softener if you are having difficulty going to the bathroom.

If lifestyle changes don't help, there are several medical treatments that can be used to shrink internal hemorrhoids. One is rubber band ligation, which involves placing a rubber band around the base of the hemorrhoid to cut off its blood supply. This will cause the hemorrhoid to shrink and eventually fall off.

Another option is sclerotherapy, which involves injecting a chemical solution into the hemorrhoid. This solution will cause the hemorrhoid to shrink.

If these treatments don't work, you may need to have surgery to remove the hemorrhoids. Surgery is typically only recommended for severe cases that haven't responded to other treatments.

If you have hemorrhoids, it's important to see your doctor so they can determine the best course of treatment for you.

How long do internal hemorrhoids take to fully heal?

Internal hemorrhoids are often not diagnosed until they cause bleeding during a bowel movement. At this point, you will need to see your doctor to find the cause of the bleeding. Internal hemorrhoids are often treated with a combination of stool softeners, added fiber to your diet, and topical creams.

In most cases, hemorrhoids will go away on their own within a few days to a couple of weeks. If your hemorrhoids do not improve with home treatment, or if they cause pain or bleeding, your doctor can treat them with special oils, creams, or suppositories. In some cases, surgery may be necessary to remove hemorrhoids.

Can internal hemorrhoids be cancerous?

Hemorrhoids are when the blood vessels in and around your anus and lower rectum become swelled and irritated. This can happen from extra pressure on these blood vessels. When you have a bowel movement, these blood vessels can swell and stretch so much that they bulge out of your anus. This is called a prolapsed hemorrhoid. Internal hemorrhoids are usually not painful but can cause bleeding when you have a bowel movement.

External hemorrhoids are the ones that can be painful because they are often irritated by your clothing or when you wipe. You can also get skin tags, which are extra skin that can form around the outside of the anus.

Prolapsed hemorrhoids can go back inside on their own or you can help them by gently pushing them back in. If they bulge out again, they may need to be removed. Hemorrhoids that cannot be pushed back in, become very swollen or bleed a lot may need to be removed with surgery.

Hemorrhoids are not cancerous. However, some of the symptoms of hemorrhoids, such as bleeding, can also be symptoms of colorectal cancer. This is why it is important to see your doctor if you have any of these symptoms.

Do internal hemorrhoids feel like poop?

Internal hemorrhoids are often described as feeling like a lump of poop that is stuck inside the rectum. The lump may be accompanied by a feeling of fullness, pressure, or pain. Many people report feeling an uncomfortable urge to have a bowel movement, even when there is no stool present. These symptoms can be mild or severe and are often worse after a bowel movement.

Internal hemorrhoids are often caused by straining during a bowel movement, pregnancy, or constipation. They can also be the result of an underlying medical condition, such as Crohn's disease or anal fistulas.

Treatment for internal hemorrhoids often includes home remedies, such as eating high-fiber foods and taking over-the-counter (OTC) medications. Some people may also need to see a doctor for more severe cases.

Surgery may be recommended for people who have large hemorrhoids that do not respond to other treatments. Surgery is also sometimes necessary if the hemorrhoids are prolapsing, or falling out of the rectum.

How do you calm an internal hemorrhoid flare up?

A hemorrhoid is an enlargement of the blood vessels in the anal or rectal area. They can be either external, coming from the anal canal, or internal, coming from the rectum. Internal hemorrhoids are usually not painful, but can bleed during a bowel movement. External hemorrhoids are often quite painful.

There are a number of things you can do to calm an internal hemorrhoid flare up. First, try to avoid constipation by eating a high fiber diet and drinking plenty of water. This will help to reduce the pressure on the hemorrhoids. If they are still bleeding, you can apply a hemorrhoidal cream or ointment to the area. This will help to soothe and protect the area.

If the hemorrhoids are extremely painful or bleeding excessively, you may need to see a doctor. In some cases, surgery may be necessary to remove the hemorrhoids. However, this is usually only necessary in severe cases.

Do internal hemorrhoids get bigger?

Internal hemorrhoids are often small, swollen veins in the wall of the anal canal.

Hemorrhoids can be painful and itchy and can sometimes bleed.

Hemorrhoids are usually the result of excess pressure on the veins in the rectum and anus.

Pregnant women are more likely to get hemorrhoids because of the extra pressure on the veins in the pelvis.

People who are overweight or who have a history of constipation are also at increased risk for hemorrhoids.

There are two types of hemorrhoids: external and internal. External hemorrhoids are usually painful and itchy and can sometimes bleed. Internal hemorrhoids are often small, swollen veins in the wall of the anal canal.

Internal hemorrhoids usually don't hurt but they can bleed.

During a bowel movement, straining can cause the veins in the hemorrhoids to bulge and rupture. This can cause bleeding.

Internal hemorrhoids can also prolapse, or protrude, through the anus. This can cause pain and irritation. prolapsed hemorrhoids can usually be pushed back into place.

Hemorrhoids are usually not a serious problem, but they can be painful and uncomfortable.

There are several things you can do to relieve the pain and discomfort of hemorrhoids:

-Take a warm sitz bath several times a day

-Apply a hemorrhoidal cream or ointment

-Use over-the-counter hemorrhoidal pads

-Take over-the-counter pain relievers, such as acetaminophen or ibuprofen

If home treatment doesn't relieve your symptoms, or if your hemorrhoids are large and very painful, you may need medical treatment.

Treatment for hemorrhoids can include:

-Rubber band ligation: A rubber band is placed around the base of the hemorrhoid to cut off its blood supply. The hemorrhoid falls off in one to two weeks.

-Sclerotherapy: A chemical solution is injected into the hemorrhoid to shrink it.

-Hemorrhoidectomy: This is surgery to remove the hemorrhoids.

Hemorrhoids are a common problem that can be very painful and annoying. Thankfully, there are many different treatments available that can help to get rid of them. If you are suffering from hemorrhoids, be sure to talk to your doctor so that you can find the best treatment for you.

Do external hemorrhoids get bigger?

External hemorrhoids are tissue swellings that form under the skin around the anus. They can be caused by straining during a bowel movement, sitting for long periods of time, or due to pregnant or giving birth. External hemorrhoids can be painful and itchy, and can sometimes crack and bleed.

While external hemorrhoids can be uncomfortable and sometimes painful, they generally do not pose a serious threat to your health. In most cases, they will go away on their own within a few days or weeks. However, if you have a large or particularly painful hemorrhoid, you may want to see a doctor for treatment.

There is no definitive answer to the question of whether or not external hemorrhoids can get bigger. In some cases, they may appear to grow larger, but this is usually just due to the swelling and inflammation associated with the condition. Once the inflammation goes down, the hemorrhoid will usually return to its original size. However, it is possible for external hemorrhoids to become more severe over time, which is why it is important to see a doctor if you are experiencing any pain or other problems with them.

What does a

n

external hemorrhoid look like?

A hemorrhoid is an enlarged vein in the anus or lower rectum. Hemorrhoids can form inside the rectum (internal hemorrhoids), or they can extend outside of the anus (external hemorrhoids). External hemorrhoids are often painful, especially if they form a blood clot. They can also itch and bleed. Internal hemorrhoids are not usually painful, but can bleed.

Hemorrhoids are very common. About half of all people have them at some point in their lives. They often occur after straining during a bowel movement, pregnancy, or childbirth. They also may occur from sitting for long periods of time on the toilet.

There are a number of things that can increase your risk of developing hemorrhoids, including:

- Straining during bowel movements

- Constipation

- Diarrhea

- Pregnancy

- Childbirth

- Sitting on the toilet for long periods of time

If you have hemorrhoids, there are a number of things you can do to relieve your symptoms:

- Take a warm bath

- Use over-the-counter creams or ointments

- Use over-the-counter medications

- Keep the area clean

If your symptoms do not improve with self-care, you may need to see a doctor. The doctor can treat hemorrhoids with medications, surgery, or other procedures.

How do I know if my external hemorrhoid is severe?

If you have an external hemorrhoid, you may be wondering how severe it is. Here are a few things to look for:

-Do you have anal pain?

-Is the hemorrhoid hard or lumpy?

-Is the hemorrhoid bleeding?

-Is the hemorrhoid enlarged?

If you have any of these symptoms, it is important to see a doctor. They will be able to determine the severity of your hemorrhoid and recommend the best course of treatment.

External hemorrhoids are often painful. If you have anal pain, it may be due to a hemorrhoid. Hemorrhoids can also bleed.Bleeding from a hemorrhoid is usually bright red. You may notice blood on toilet paper after having a bowel movement. Blood can also be found in the toilet bowl.

Hemorrhoids can also become enlarged. An enlarged hemorrhoid can prolapse, or protrude, through the anus. Prolapsed hemorrhoids can be very painful. They can also lead to bleeding.

If you have any of these symptoms, it is important to see a doctor. They will be able to determine the severity of your hemorrhoid and recommend the best course of treatment.

Does walking help hemorrhoids?

It is a common belief that Walking is a good exercise to relieve hemorrhoids but is it really effective?

There are two types of hemorrhoids, external and internal. Internal hemorrhoids are located inside the anal canal while external hemorrhoids are found under the skin around the anus. Both types of hemorrhoids can be painful and cause bleeding.

Walking is a good exercise for overall health but it is not clear if it is effective for relieving hemorrhoids. One study found that walking was not effective for relieving symptoms of hemorrhoids. However, the study was small and more research is needed to confirm these results.

Home

remedies to relieve symptoms

•

If you have hemorrhoids, you can try different home remedies to relieve symptoms. Some home remedies include:

- Eating high-fiber foods to soften stools and reduce constipation

- Drinking plenty of fluids to prevent dehydration

- Applying a hemorrhoid cream or ointment to the affected area

You can also talk to your doctor about medical treatment options for hemorrhoids. Some treatment options include:

- Rubber band ligation: A rubber band is placed around the base of the hemorrhoid to cut off the blood supply. The hemorrhoid then falls off after a few days.

- Sclerotherapy: A chemical solution is injected around the blood vessels to shrink the hemorrhoids.

- Infrared coagulation: A device is used to apply heat to the blood vessels to shrink the hemorrhoids.

If you are struggling with hemorrhoids, it is important to talk to your doctor to find the best treatment option for you.

How do you shrink piles completely?

There is no one-size-fits-all answer to how to shrink piles completely, as the best way to do so will vary depending on the individual and the severity of their hemorrhoids. However, there are a few things that anyone looking to shrink their piles should keep in mind.

First and foremost, it is important to keep the area clean and free from irritants. This means gently cleansing the area with warm water after each bowel movement, and avoiding the use of harsh soaps or wipes. It is also important to pat the area dry, rather than rubbing it, to avoid further irritation.

Secondly, it is important to avoid constipation and straining during bowel movements. This can be done by eating a high-fiber diet and staying hydrated. Taking a stool softener or laxative may also be necessary.

Finally, there are a number of topical treatments that can be used to help shrink hemorrhoids. These include over-the-counter creams and ointments, as well as home remedies like witch hazel or aloe vera. In more severe cases, your doctor may recommend surgery to remove the hemorrhoids.

How long does it take for piles to heal naturally?

Piles, also known as hemorrhoids, are swollen veins in the anal and rectal area. They can be painful and itchy, and can sometimes bleed. If you have piles, you may be wondering how long it will take for them to heal.

There are different types of piles, and they can vary in how long it takes for them to heal. Internal piles are usually the most uncomfortable, but they can often be treated with over-the-counter medications. External piles can be more painful, and may require prescription-strength creams or ointments.

In most cases, piles will go away on their own within a few days to a couple of weeks. If you have severe piles, however, they may take longer to heal. If your piles are not improving after a couple of weeks, or if they are becoming more painful, you should see a doctor.

There are several things you can do to help speed up the healing process. Avoiding constipation can be helpful, as this can make piles worse. Eating a high-fiber diet and drinking plenty of fluids can help to keep you regular. You can also try using over-the-counter hemorrhoid creams or ointments.

If your piles are severe, your doctor may recommend a hemorrhoidectomy, which is a surgical procedure to remove the piles. This is usually only recommended for severe cases that have not responded to other treatment methods.

Most people will not need surgery and can treat their piles at home. With proper care, most piles will heal within a few days to weeks.

If you're experiencing hemorrhoids, you're not alone. Hemorrhoids are a common condition, especially among adults aged 45 to 65. There are two main types of hemorrhoids: internal and external. Internal hemorrhoids are located inside the rectum, while external hemorrhoids develop around the anus. Hemorrhoids can be painful and irritating, but they're typically not serious. In most cases, hemorrhoids can be treated at home with over-the-counter creams, ointments, and medicated wipes. If home treatment doesn't work, your doctor may recommend a minimally invasive procedure to remove the hemorrhoids.

When should I go to the doctor for internal hemorrhoids?

If you have hemorrhoids, you may not need to see a doctor. Hemorrhoids are common and usually clear up on their own without treatment.

You should see a doctor if your hemorrhoids bleed a lot, hurt a lot, or if you are having a hard time going to the bathroom. Also, see a doctor if you have hemorrhoids that come out of your anus all the time. These are called prolapsed hemorrhoids.

If you have any of these problems, the doctor will look at your anus and rectum. The doctor may also do a digital rectal exam. This is where the doctor puts a gloved finger in your anus to check for bleeding or anything else that may be wrong.

If the doctor thinks you have hemorrhoids, they may do a sigmoidoscopy. This is a test where they put a small, flexible tube with a light in your anus and rectum. They use this to look for bleeding or anything else that may be wrong.

If the doctor thinks you have hemorrhoids, they may do a colonoscopy. This is a test where they put a long, flexible tube with a light in your anus and rectum. They use this to look at your entire colon.

You may need surgery if your hemorrhoids are very large and do not go away with home treatment. Hemorrhoid surgery is called a hemorrhoidectomy.

How common are internal hemorrhoids?

Hemorrhoids are swollen blood vessels in the lower part of the rectum or anus. They usually occur when the blood vessels around the anus or rectum become swollen or dilated. Hemorrhoids can be either internal, meaning they are inside the rectum or anus, or external, meaning they are outside the rectum or anus.

Internal hemorrhoids are more common than external hemorrhoids. They usually don't cause discomfort because the rectum and anus have few pain-sensing nerves. External hemorrhoids, on the other hand, are covered with a thin layer of skin and have many pain-sensing nerves. This is why external hemorrhoids can be painful.

There are a number of things that can cause hemorrhoids, including:

- Constipation: This is one of the most common causes of hemorrhoids. When you are constipated, you have to strain a lot to have a bowel movement. This straining can cause the blood vessels in your anus or rectum to become swollen or dilated.

- Pregnancy: This is another common cause of hemorrhoids. During pregnancy, the growing uterus puts extra pressure on the blood vessels in the pelvic area. This can cause the vessels to become swollen or dilated.

- Anal intercourse: This can also cause the blood vessels in the anus or rectum to become swollen or dilated.

- Age: As people get older, the tissues that support the blood vessels in the anus and rectum can become weak and stretch out. This can cause the vessels to become more swollen or dilated.

There are a number of things you can do to prevent hemorrhoids. Some of these include:

- Eat a high-fiber diet: This will help you avoid constipation, which can lead to hemorrhoids.

- Avoid sitting for long periods of time: This can put extra pressure on the blood vessels in your anus or rectum and cause them to become swollen or dilated.

- Exercise: This can help to improve the circulation in your pelvis and help to prevent hemorrhoids.

If you do develop hemorrhoids, there are a number of things you can do to treat them. Some of these include:

- Use over-the-counter creams or ointments: This can help to soothe the pain and itching associated with hemorrhoids.

- Take a sitz bath: This is a special type of bath that can help to reduce swelling and pain.

- Use stool softeners: This can help to reduce constipation and straining, which can worsen hemorrhoids.

Hemorrhoids are relatively common, especially among people over the age of 50. If you have hemorrhoids, there are a number of things you can do to treat them and relieve the discomfort they can cause.

What do inflamed internal hemorrhoids feel like?

Hemorrhoids are often described as feeling like a lump or bulge near the anus. They may be itchy or painful, and can sometimes bleed. This can happen when they become inflamed or swollen.

When hemorrhoids become inflamed, they can feel a variety of different ways. Some people describe the feeling as a sharp pain, while others say it feels more like a burning sensation. It is not uncommon for the area to feel sore or tender to the touch.

The sensation of having hemorrhoids can vary depending on the individual and the severity of the inflammation. For some people, the feeling may only be noticed when they are sitting down or having a bowel movement. Others may feel the discomfort all the time.

If you are dealing with inflamed hemorrhoids, there are a few things you can do to help ease the discomfort. Applying a hemorrhoid cream or ointment to the area can help soothe the skin. You can also take a sitz bath, which is a type of bath that allows you to soak the area in warm water.

If you are experiencing pain or discomfort from your hemorrhoids, it is important to talk to your doctor. They can help you determine the best course of treatment and make sure that your symptoms are not indicative of a more serious condition.

There are a few different things that people can do in order to treat hemorrhoids. For example, people can use over-the-counter creams, take sitz baths, or use stool softeners. However, if hemorrhoids are severe, people may need to see a doctor.

Do you need a colonoscopy to check for internal hemorrhoids?

A colonoscopy is a diagnostic procedure that allows a doctor to look at the entire colon and find any abnormal growths or changes. This includes internal hemorrhoids.

Internal hemorrhoids are veins that have become inflamed and swollen within the lower rectum and anus. These veins can become so large that they protrude from the anus. Internal hemorrhoids can be very painful and may require treatment.

A colonoscopy is the best way to definitively diagnose internal hemorrhoids. During a colonoscopy, a doctor can directly visualize the hemorrhoids and any other abnormalities in the colon. This allows for a more accurate diagnosis and can help rule out other potential causes of symptoms.

If you are experiencing symptoms that may be due to internal hemorrhoids, such as rectal bleeding, pain, or itching, it is important to see a doctor for a diagnosis. Your doctor may recommend a colonoscopy to confirm the diagnosis and rule out other potential causes of your symptoms.

What happens if you have hemorrhoids for years?

Can hemorrhoids go away on their own?

If you have hemorrhoids for an extended period of time, they may not go away on their own. In this case, you would need to seek medical attention in order to have them removed. However, there are some things you can do at home to help ease the discomfort caused by hemorrhoids.

For one, you can try to soak the area in warm water for 20 minutes each day. This can help to soothe the area and reduce inflammation. You can also try using over-the-counter creams or ointments to help with the pain and discomfort.

If you find that your hemorrhoids are becoming more painful or are interfering with your daily activities, it is important to see a doctor. They can prescribe stronger medications or recommend a procedure to remove the hemorrhoids.

It is important to keep in mind that hemorrhoids are generally not a serious condition and can often be treated at home. However, if you are experiencing severe pain, bleeding, or other problems, it is important to see a doctor so that they can rule out other potential causes.

How do you get rid of hemorrhoids external?

There is no one definitive answer to this question, as there are several ways that people have found to be effective in treating hemorrhoids externally. Some common methods include:

- Soaking the affected area in warm water for several minutes at a time. This can help to soothe the irritation and pain associated with hemorrhoids.

- Applying a topical cream or ointment specifically designed to relieve hemorrhoid symptoms.

- Taking over-the-counter medication such as ibuprofen or acetaminophen to help reduce pain and inflammation.

- avoiding sitting or standing for long periods of time, as this can aggravate hemorrhoids.

- Eating a high-fiber diet and drinking plenty of fluids to help soften stool and reduce constipation, which can cause or worsen hemorrhoids.

- Exercising regularly to help reduce pressure on the veins in the rectal and anal area.

If home treatment measures are not providing relief, or if the hemorrhoids are large and painful, you may need to see a doctor for further treatment options. Procedures that can be done to treat hemorrhoids externally include:

- Rubber band ligation, in which a rubber band is placed around the base of the hemorrhoid to cut off its blood supply.

- Sclerotherapy, in which a chemical solution is injected around the blood vessels of the hemorrhoid to shrink it.

- Infrared coagulation, in which a device is used to deliver infrared light to the blood vessels of the hemorrhoid to destroy them.

- Hemorrhoidectomy, in which the hemorrhoid is surgically removed.

You should always consult with a medical professional before pursuing any treatment option for hemorrhoids, as they can help to determine which method is right for you based on the severity of your condition.

Do external

hemorrh

o

ids

go away?

External hemorrhoids are often large, sore, and uncomfortable. But they usually don't last long. In most cases, they go away on their own in a week or two.

Here's what you can do to relieve the pain and help them heal:

- Take over-the-counter pain relievers like ibuprofen or aspirin.

- Apply an over-the-counter cream or ointment to the area. A 1% hydrocortisone cream applied to the area can help reduce pain and swelling.

- Soak in a warm tub for 15 minutes a few times a day.

- Don't strain or hold your breath when you go to the bathroom. This puts extra pressure on the veins in your anus and can make hemorrhoids worse.

- Try taking a stool softener, such as psyllium husk, to make it easier to go.
- Don't sit on the toilet for more than a few minutes. This can make hemorrhoids worse.

If home treatments aren't helping, or if your hemorrhoids are bleeding, see your doctor. They may be able to prescribe a stronger cream or medicine. In some cases, surgery may be necessary to remove hemorrhoids.

This FAQ has provided an overview of hemorrhoids, their causes, and treatments. Despite their often embarrassing and uncomfortable symptoms, hemorrhoids are a common condition that is usually not serious. With proper care, they can often be treated at home. If you are experiencing symptoms of hemorrhoids, talk to your doctor to determine the best course of treatment for you.

What can aggravate internal hemorrhoids?

There are a number of things that can aggravate internal hemorrhoids, including straining during bowel movements, sitting for long periods of time, and lifting heavy objects. Other activities that can aggravate internal hemorrhoids include coughing, sneezing, and pregnancy.

Straining during bowel movements is one of the most common activities that can aggravate internal hemorrhoids. This is because straining puts unnecessary pressure on the veins in the anal area, which can cause them to become swollen and inflamed. If you are prone to hemorrhoids, it is important to make sure you are using the bathroom properly. This means going when you first feel the urge, and not holding it in. It is also important to avoid straining by using a stool softener if necessary, and by taking a seat on the toilet rather than squatting.

Sitting for long periods of time can also aggravate internal hemorrhoids. This is because when you sit, there is more pressure placed on the veins in your anal area. This pressure can cause the veins to become swollen and inflamed. If you have a desk job or you are required to sit for long periods of time, it is important to take breaks every so often to walk around and stretch. Additionally, you may want to consider using a hemorrhoid pillow to relieve some of the pressure on your veins.

Lifting heavy objects can also aggravate internal hemorrhoids. This is because lifting puts additional pressure on the veins in the anal area. If you must lift heavy objects, it is important to use proper lifting technique. This means using your legs to lift rather than your back, and avoiding any sudden or jerking motions.

Coughing, sneezing, and pregnancy can also aggravate internal hemorrhoids. This is because these activities put additional pressure on the veins in the anal area. If you are pregnant, it is important to talk to your doctor about ways to reduce the pressure on your veins. Additionally, if you are prone to hemorrhoids, it is important to take care when coughing or sneezing. You may want to cover your mouth and nose with a tissue to avoid putting unnecessary pressure on your veins.

Do internal hemorrhoids get inflamed?

Internal hemorrhoids are often not as painful as external hemorrhoids because the swollen tissue is not in direct contact with anal nerves. However, internal hemorrhoids may bleed, and the blood can be visible in the stool or on toilet paper. If bleeding is severe, you may see blood in the toilet bowl.

Internal hemorrhoids are graded according to their level of protrusion into the anal canal. Grade 1 and 2 hemorrhoids protrude into the canal but do not prolapse, or bulge, outside of the anal opening. Grade 3 hemorrhoids protrude from the anal opening and prolapse outside the body during a bowel movement but spontaneously return inside the anal canal afterward. Grade 4 hemorrhoids are permanently prolapsed and cannot be manually pushed back into the anal canal.

Symptoms of internal hemorrhoids may include:

- bleeding when having a bowel movement

- anal itching

- pain or discomfort, especially when sitting

Internal hemorrhoids can become inflamed and very painful when the swollen tissue is irritated or damaged. Thrombosed hemorrhoids occur when an internal hemorrhoid develops a blood clot, which can cause severe pain, inflammation, and swelling.

If you have any symptoms of internal hemorrhoids, see your doctor for a proper diagnosis and treatment. hemorrhoids are usually treated with dietary changes, over-the-counter (OTC) creams and ointments, and home remedies. In more severe cases, hemorrhoids may require more aggressive treatment, such as rubber band ligation, sclerotherapy, infrared coagulation, or surgery.

Internal hemorrhoids are often not as painful as external hemorrhoids because the swollen tissue is not in direct contact with anal nerves. However, internal hemorrhoids may bleed, and the blood can be visible in the stool or on toilet paper. If bleeding is severe, you may see blood in the toilet bowl.

Internal hemorrhoids are graded according to their level of protrusion into the anal canal. Grade 1 and 2 hemorrhoids protrude into the canal but do not prolapse, or bulge, outside of the anal opening. Grade 3 hemorrhoids protrude from the anal opening and prolapse outside the body during a bowel movement but spontaneously return inside the anal canal afterward. Grade 4 hemorrhoids are permanently prolapsed and cannot be manually pushed back into the anal canal.

Symptoms of internal hemorrhoids may include:

- bleeding when having a bowel movement

- anal itching

- pain or discomfort, especially when sitting

Internal hemorrhoids can become inflamed and very painful when the swollen tissue is irritated or damaged. Thrombosed hemorrhoids occur when an internal hemorrhoid develops a blood clot, which can cause severe pain, inflammation, and swelling.

If you have any symptoms of internal hemorrhoids, see your doctor for a proper diagnosis and

Can doctors do anything for internal hemorrhoids?

Hemorrhoids are a common condition that can cause a lot of pain and discomfort. They are usually caused by sitting or standing for long periods of time, or from straining during bowel movements. Hemorrhoids can be internal or external, and typically, internal hemorrhoids are more painful. There are a few different ways that doctors can treat hemorrhoids, depending on the severity of the condition.

For mild hemorrhoids, doctors may recommend over the counter creams or ointments to help with the pain and discomfort. Heating pads or Sitz baths (where you sit in a few inches of warm water) can also help. If these home treatments don't work, or if the hemorrhoids are more severe, then doctors can do a number of different procedures.

One common procedure is called rubber band ligation. This is where the doctor puts a special rubber band around the base of the hemorrhoid. This cuts off the blood supply to the hemorrhoid and eventually, it will fall off. This is typically a very effective procedure with minimal pain.

Another common procedure is called sclerotherapy. This is where the doctor injects a chemical solution into the hemorrhoid. This solution makes the blood vessels swell and the hemorrhoid will shrink.

For more severe hemorrhoids, doctors may recommend surgery. This is usually a last resort, but it is sometimes necessary. The most common surgery for hemorrhoids is called hemorrhoidectomy. This is where the doctor removes the hemorrhoids.

There are a number of different ways to treat hemorrhoids, and the best option will depend on the severity of the condition. If home treatments are not working, or if the hemorrhoids are more severe, then doctors can do a number of different procedures.

Can a GP diagnose internal hemorrhoids?

A GP can diagnose internal hemorrhoids by taking a medical history and performing a physical examination. The physical examination may include a digital rectal examination, which involves the GPinserting a lubricated, gloved finger into the rectum to feel for any lumps or abnormalities. If the GP suspects that the person has internal hemorrhoids, they may refer them to a specialist for further testing.

Internal hemorrhoids are often not painful, but they can cause bleeding. The most common symptom of internal hemorrhoids is bright red blood on the toilet paper or in the toilet bowl after a bowel movement. Other symptoms may include bleeding from the anus, itching or irritation in the anal area, and a feeling of fullness in the rectum.

If you have any of these symptoms, it is important to see your GP so that they can rule out other potential causes, such as anal fissures, anal fistulas, or colorectal cancer.

Does walking shrink hemorrhoids?

There are a few things that can help shrink hemorrhoids fast. Walking is one of them. Walking keeps things moving in your digestive system, which can help reduce the chances of constipation, a major cause of hemorrhoids. Even just a brief walk around the block can be helpful.

If you have hemorrhoids, you may be tempted to stay home and not move around much. But that's actually the worst thing you can do. Activity helps keep things moving in your digestive system and can help reduce the chances of constipation, a major cause of hemorrhoids. Walking is a great form of exercise for people with hemorrhoids. Even just a brief walk around the block can be helpful.

If you have hemorrhoids, you may be noticing them more now that you're spending more time at home. That's because activity helps keep things moving in your digestive system, and can help reduce the chances of constipation, a major cause of hemorrhoids. Walking is a great form of exercise for people with hemorrhoids. Even just a brief walk around the block can be helpful.

So, if you're looking for ways to shrink hemorrhoids fast, remember that walking is one of the best things you can do. Just a brief walk around the block can be helpful. So get up and move!

How to treat hemorrhoids is a question many people ask themselves when they find out they have this common condition. Hemorrhoids are swollen blood vessels in the anal area. They can be very painful, itchy and bleed. Home remedies, over the counter treatments and surgery are all options for treating hemorrhoids.

Should I be worried if I keep getting hemorrhoids?

If you are frequently getting hemorrhoids, it is important to consult with a doctor to rule out any other underlying conditions. While hemorrhoids are generally not serious, they can be a sign of other problems. If you are experiencing any pain, bleeding, or discomfort from your hemorrhoids, it is important to see a doctor to get a proper diagnosis and treatment plan.

Can dehydration cause hemorrhoids?

Dehydration can cause hemorrhoids for a number of reasons. When a person is dehydrated, the body's tissues and organs do not have enough fluid to function properly. This can cause the blood vessels to constrict and the stool to become hard and dry, making it difficult to pass. This can lead to increased pressure on the veins in the rectum and anus, which can cause them to swell and bleed. In addition, dehydration can also reduce the body's production of mucus, which lubricates and softens the stool, making it easier to pass.

Dehydration is a common problem, especially in people who are ill, have diarrhoea or are vomiting. It can also be caused by not drinking enough fluids or by sweating a lot. Symptoms of dehydration include feeling thirsty, having a dry mouth, feeling tired, having dark urine and feeling dizzy. If you are dehydrated, it is important to drink plenty of fluids, such as water or an electrolyte-containing drink. You should also seek medical help if you have severe dehydration or if you are unable to keep fluids down.

Dehydration is a common cause of constipation, which can in turn lead to hemorrhoids. In order to avoid hemorrhoids, it is important to stay hydrated by drinking plenty of fluids and eating a high-fiber diet. If you are already constipated, you should try to soften your stool by drinking more fluids and eating foods that are high in fiber. If you are unable to relieve constipation with these measures, you should see a doctor.

Does coffee make hemorrhoids worse?

Dr. Tan Hoong Wei says that there is no evidence that coffee makes hemorrhoids worse. In fact, a cup of coffee may even help relieve constipation, which can be a contributing factor to hemorrhoids. decaffeinated coffee is just as effective as regular coffee.

Coffee is not the only beverage that can relieve constipation. Other options include prune juice, water, and herbal teas.

What foods heal hemorrhoids?

Hemorrhoids are a common and painful affliction. They are often caused by constipation, straining during bowel movements, and sitting for long periods of time on the toilet. Hemorrhoids can also be caused by pregnancy, being overweight, and other factors.

There are several foods that can help to heal hemorrhoids. These include:

-Fiber-rich foods: Eating plenty of fiber-rich foods, such as fruits, vegetables, whole grains, and beans, can help to soften stools and reduce constipation, which can help to heal hemorrhoids.

-Sitz baths: Soaking the affected area in a sitz bath (a shallow basin of warm water) for 15-20 minutes several times a day can help to reduce pain and swelling.

-Ice: Applying ice to the affected area can help to reduce pain and swelling.

-Hemorrhoid cream: Applying hemorrhoid cream to the affected area can also help to reduce pain and swelling.

Making lifestyle changes, such as eating a high-fiber diet, drinking plenty of water, and exercising regularly, can also help to prevent hemorrhoids from developing in the first place.

Do internal hemorrhoids need colonoscopy?

The chances of developing hemorrhoids increase as people get older. Internal hemorrhoids are often not noticed until they bleed. When this happens, it is usually during and after a bowel movement. The blood may be bright red and cover the stool, or it may be on toilet paper or in the toilet bowl. A person with hemorrhoids may also feel discomfort, itching, or pain around the anus.

Hemorrhoids are commonly treated with over-the-counter medication, according to the Mayo Clinic. Some people may need surgery if the hemorrhoids are large and not responding to other treatments.

A colonoscopy is not typically needed to treat internal hemorrhoids, unless they are severe and bleeding. If a person has rectal bleeding that is not from hemorrhoids, a colonoscopy may be done to rule out other causes, such as colorectal cancer.

Hemorrhoids are a common and often painful condition caused by swollen blood vessels in the anus and rectum. Although hemorrhoids can be embarrassing and uncomfortable, they are usually not a serious health problem. However, if the hemorrhoids bleed a lot, become too big, or are extremely painful, you should see your doctor. There are a number of treatments that can help relieve the symptoms of hemorrhoids.

Are external hemorrhoids serious?

Most people with hemorrhoids experience only mild symptoms, and external hemorrhoids are no exception. In most cases, they will go away on their own within a few days. However, if you experience more severe symptoms, such as intense pain, bleeding, or prolapse, then you should see a doctor. External hemorrhoids can sometimes be serious, but this is usually only the case if they become prolapsed or thrombosed.

Prolapsed hemorrhoids are those that bulge out from the anus. This can happen if they become too large or they are not treated properly. If prolapse occurs, it is important to see a doctor, as it can be quite painful. Prolapsed hemorrhoids may also bleed.

Thrombosed hemorrhoids are those that have a blood clot within them. This can happen if the hemorrhoid becomes irritated or damaged. Thrombosed hemorrhoids can be very painful, and they may also bleed. If you have a thrombosed hemorrhoid, it is important to see a doctor so that the clot can be removed.

External hemorrhoids are usually not serious, but they can sometimes cause problems. If you experience any severe symptoms, it is important to see a doctor so that they can be treated properly.

How long does an external hemorrhoid last?

External hemorrhoids are a lot like internal hemorrhoids, only they bulge outwards from the anus instead of bulging into the rectum. They can be very painful, especially if they get thrombosed, or full of blood. They can itch, bleed, and make sitting or going to the bathroom very uncomfortable.

So, how long do external hemorrhoids last? Just like internal hemorrhoids, they can last for days, weeks, or even months. The good news is that, unlike internal hemorrhoids, they can be treated with over-the-counter ointments, creams, or suppositories. The bad news is that, because they are on the outside, they can get irritated and inflamed more easily, which can make them even more painful.

If you have an external hemorrhoid that is causing you a lot of pain, you should see a doctor. They can prescribe you a stronger cream or ointment to help with the pain, or they can even do a minor surgery to remove the hemorrhoid. In most cases, though, external hemorrhoids will go away on their own eventually.

What is the fastest way to get rid of external hemorrhoids?

Hemorrhoids are one of the most common and nagging medical conditions. They are also one of the most misunderstood. Many people think they are just a nuisance, but they can be quite painful and even disabling.

The good news is that there are several hundred treatment options available for hemorrhoids, ranging from home remedies to surgery. The best way to determine the best course of treatment for you is to consult with a medical professional.

There are two types of hemorrhoids: external and internal. External hemorrhoids are located outside of the rectum and are usually visible. Internal hemorrhoids are located inside the rectum and are not usually visible.

The most common symptom of hemorrhoids is bleeding during bowel movements. Other symptoms include itching, pain, and swelling.

There are several things you can do to treat hemorrhoids at home. These include:

- Taking over-the-counter pain medication such as ibuprofen or aspirin

- Applying a topical cream or ointment such as hydrocortisone

- Soaking the area in warm water for 10-15 minutes

- Avoiding sitting or standing for long periods of time

If home remedies don't work, there are a number of other treatment options available. These include:

- Rubber band ligation: A rubber band is placed around the base of the hemorrhoid to cut off its blood supply. The hemorrhoid then falls off in a week or two.

- Sclerotherapy: A chemical solution is injected into the hemorrhoid to shrink it.

- Infrared coagulation: A device is used to deliver a burst of infrared light to the hemorrhoid, which causes it to shrink.

- Hemorrhoidectomy: This is surgery to remove the hemorrhoid. It is usually only done for very large hemorrhoids.

The best way to prevent hemorrhoids is to avoid constipation. To do this, you should:

- Eat a diet that is high in fiber

- Drink plenty of fluids

- Exercise regularly

- Avoid sitting or standing for long periods of time

Should I be worried about an external hemorrhoid?

If you have an external hemorrhoid, you may be concerned about it. Here are a few things to keep in mind:

-External hemorrhoids are usually not painful, but they can cause bleeding.

-If you have an external hemorrhoid, you may be able to see or feel it.

-External hemorrhoids are not usually dangerous, but they can be uncomfortable.

-If you have an external hemorrhoid that is causing bleeding or pain, you should see a doctor.

External hemorrhoids are usually not a cause for concern. However, if you have one that is causing bleeding or pain, you should see a doctor.

When it comes to hemorrhoids, it is important to know all of the facts. hemorrhoids can be a very embarrassing and painful problem, but luckily, there are many treatments available. With the right treatment, hemorrhoids can be quickly and easily resolved.

Can you naturally get rid of external hemorrhoids?

External hemorrhoids are a common and painful problem. Many people try different methods to get rid of them, but they often come back. You may be able to find relief from your symptoms by using home treatments.

Surgery is sometimes needed to remove hemorrhoids. But even if you have surgery, hemorrhoids can come back. You can help lower your chance of getting hemorrhoids again by making lifestyle changes. These include eating a high-fiber diet, avoiding constipation, and not straining when you have a bowel movement.

You can also help prevent hemorrhoids by not sitting on the toilet for long periods of time. And don't hold your breath when you're having a bowel movement. This can make the hemorrhoids worse.

How to shrink external hemorrhoids naturally fast and easy?

Hemorrhoids are a common condition that affects millions of people worldwide. They are caused by inflammation of the veins in the anal or rectal area and can be either internal or external. Internal hemorrhoids are usually not painful, but can bleed. External hemorrhoids are usually painful and can cause bleeding.

There are several ways to shrink hemorrhoids naturally fast and easy. These include:

1. Sitz baths.

Sitz baths are a great way to reduce the swelling and inflammation of hemorrhoids. simply sit in a tub of warm water for about 15 minutes. This will help to soothe the anal area and reduce the pain and discomfort associated with hemorrhoids.

2. Exercise.

Exercise is important for overall health, but it can also help to reduce the size of hemorrhoids. Exercise helps to increase blood flow and reduce the pressure on the veins in the anal area. This can help to reduce the inflammation and swelling of hemorrhoids.

3. Diet.

Eating a healthy diet is important for overall health, but it can also help to reduce the size of hemorrhoids. Eating a diet that is high in fiber can help to reduce the chances of constipation, which can worsen hemorrhoids. Fiber can also help to soften stool, which can make it easier to pass and reduce the discomfort associated with hemorrhoids.

4. Supplements.

There are a number of supplements that can help to reduce the size of hemorrhoids. These include witch hazel, butcher's broom, and horse chestnut. These supplements can help to reduce the inflammation and swelling of hemorrhoids.

5. Creams and ointments.

There are a number of over the counter creams and ointments that can help to shrink hemorrhoids. These include Preparation H, Hemorrhoidal, and Anusol. These products can help to soothe the anal area and reduce the pain and discomfort associated with hemorrhoids.

This FAQ discusses hemorrhoids, which are a common and painful problem. There are many home remedies and treatments available. With proper treatment, most people can get relief from their symptoms.

How do you treat internal hemorrhoids?

There are many ways to treat internal hemorrhoids, depending on the severity of the condition. For mild hemorrhoids, over-the-counter creams and ointments can be effective in reducing irritation and pain. More severe cases may require prescription medication, and in some cases, surgery may be necessary to remove the hemorrhoids.

For milder cases of internal hemorrhoids, over-the-counter hemorrhoid creams and ointments can provide relief from pain and irritation. These products typically contain ingredients like George or hydrocortisone that can reduce inflammation. It is important to read the labels carefully and follow the directions for use to avoid further irritation of the area.

If over-the-counter products do not provide enough relief, hemorrhoid creams and ointments that are available by prescription may be more effective. These products typically contain stronger active ingredients than their over-the-counter counterparts. Again, it is important to follow the directions for use to avoid further irritation or damage to the area.

In some cases, surgery may be necessary to remove internal hemorrhoids. This is typically only recommended for severe cases that have not responded to other treatment methods. Surgery may involve removal of the hemorrhoids themselves, or it may involve correction of an underlying condition that is causing the hemorrhoids.

No matter what treatment method is used, it is important to drink plenty of fluids and eat a high-fiber diet to avoid constipation. This can help to reduce the pressure on the hemorrhoids and make them less likely to become irritated or inflamed. If you are experiencing severe pain or bleeding, please see a doctor for evaluation and treatment.

Do internal hemorrhoids go away?

Internal hemorrhoids can be quite painful, making it difficult to sit down, stand up, or have a bowel movement. They can also bleed, which can be quite alarming. The good news is that, in most cases, internal hemorrhoids will go away on their own.

There are a few things you can do to speed up the process and help relieve the pain in the meantime. Taking a warm bath can help soothe the area and promote healing. You can also use a medicated cream or ointment to help with the pain and inflammation. If the hemorrhoids are particularly large or painful, your doctor may recommend a minimally-invasive procedure to remove them.

In most cases, internal hemorrhoids will go away on their own within a few days to a week. If they don't, or if they keep coming back, you should see your doctor for further evaluation.

If you have hemorrhoids, you may be feeling embarrassed, uncomfortable, and in pain. But you're not alone—hemorrhoids are a very common condition. In fact, about 75 percent of Americans will experience hemorrhoids at least once in their lives.

There are two types of hemorrhoids: internal and external. Internal hemorrhoids are located inside the rectum, and external hemorrhoids are located under the skin around the anus. Hemorrhoids are usually caused by straining during bowel movements, pregnancy, and childbirth.

There are a number of treatments for hemorrhoids, including over-the-counter creams and ointments, suppositories, and sitz baths. In some cases, surgery may be necessary.

No matter what treatment you choose, hemorrhoids can be a painful and frustrating condition. But with the help of your doctor, you can find relief.

Do hemorrhoids cause gas?

Hemorrhoids are often thought of as a minor nuisance, but they can cause major discomfort. Hemorrhoids are swollen veins in the anal canal. They can be internal, which means they're inside the rectum. Or they can be external, which means they're under the skin around the anus. Either way, when they swell, they can cause a variety of symptoms.

People often ask if hemorrhoids cause gas. The answer is yes, hemorrhoids can cause gas. Hemorrhoids can block the anal opening, which can lead to gas and bloating. Hemorrhoids can also be very painful, and the pain can make it difficult to have a bowel movement. This can also lead to gas and bloating.

There are a few things you can do to ease the gas and bloating if you have hemorrhoids. First, try to go to the bathroom as soon as you feel the urge. This can help prevent constipation, which can make gas and bloating worse. Second, eat a high-fiber diet. This can help keep things moving through your digestive system, making it less likely that gas will build up. Third, try to avoid foods that are known to cause gas. These include fatty foods, processed foods, dairy products, and beans. And finally, if you're still struggling with gas and bloating, talk to your doctor. They can prescribe medication that can help relieve the symptoms.

Does IBS cause hemorrhoids?

There is no one-size-fits-all answer to this question, as the relationship between IBS and hemorrhoids may vary from person to person. However, it is worth noting that both conditions can cause similar symptoms, such as abdominal pain, bloating, and constipation. For this reason, it is not uncommon for people with IBS to also experience hemorrhoids.

There are a number of possible explanations for the link between IBS and hemorrhoids. One theory is that both conditions may be associated with changes in the gut microbiota. Alterations in gut microbiota have been linked to a number of gastrointestinal conditions, including IBS and hemorrhoids. Another possibility is that IBS and hemorrhoids may share a common underlying cause, such as inflammation or nerve dysfunction.

In some cases, hemorrhoids may also be a symptom of IBS. This is known as "inflammatory bowel-related anal disease" (IBRAD). IBRAD is a condition that is characterized by inflammation of the anal area. Symptoms of IBRAD can include anal bleeding, pain, and itching. While IBS and IBRAD are not the same condition, they can share similar features.

If you are experiencing symptoms of IBS and hemorrhoids, it is important to see a healthcare provider for a proper diagnosis. They will be able to rule out other potential causes of your symptoms and determine the best course of treatment.

If you have hemorrhoids, there are a few things you can do to relieve the pain. You can try over-the-counter creams and ointments, use ice packs, or take oral pain relievers. If home remedies don't work, your doctor can prescribe medication. In some cases, surgery may be necessary.

Can internal hemorrhoids last for months?

Internal hemorrhoids are often associated with painless bleeding. However, they can cause severe pain if they prolapse, or bulge, from the anus. If prolapse occurs, it may be necessary to reduce, or push, the hemorrhoid back into place. A prolapsed hemorrhoid may develop a blood clot, which can lead to severe pain and swelling. Internal hemorrhoids may also be associated with anal fissures, or small tears in the anal canal.

Internal hemorrhoids can last for months, and may eventually require surgical intervention. If you have internal hemorrhoids, it is important to see a doctor if you experience any rectal bleeding, as this could be a sign of a more serious condition. Internal hemorrhoids are usually diagnosed with a physical examination and a medical history. If prolapse is suspected, a rectal exam may be performed.

Many people experience hemorrhoids at some point in their lives. They are usually not serious and can be treated with over-the-counter creams or ointments. However, if hemorrhoids are severe or recurrent, you may need to see a doctor for treatment.

How serious are internal hemorrhoids?

Internal hemorrhoids are usually small veins located in the lining of the rectum or anus. These veins can become swollen and cause discomfort, particularly when passing stool. Internal hemorrhoids are usually not painful unless they protrude through the anal opening, in which case they can cause pain and bleeding.

In most cases, internal hemorrhoids are mild and do not require treatment. However, if they are large and cause significant bleeding or pain, they may need to be treated. There are a number of treatment options available, including rubber band ligation, in which a rubber band is placed around the base of the hemorrhoid to cut off its blood supply; sclerotherapy, in which a chemical solution is injected into the hemorrhoid to shrink it; and surgery.

Internal hemorrhoids are typically not a serious condition, but they can be painful and uncomfortable. If you are experiencing any symptoms, talk to your doctor to find the best treatment option for you.

What happens if internal hemorrhoids go untreated?

If internal hemorrhoids go untreated, they can cause a number of problems. One of the most serious is bleeding. When the hemorrhoids are swollen, they can put pressure on the blood vessels in the anal area and cause them to break. This can lead to bleeding from the anus, which can be severe.

Another potential problem is prolapse. This is when the hemorrhoids become so large and swollen that they actually push through the anus. This can be extremely painful and can make it difficult to have a bowel movement.

If prolapse occurs, it is important to see a doctor right away. If left untreated, prolapse can lead to tissue death in the area. This can create an opening in the anal canal, which can allow bacteria to enter the bloodstream and cause serious infections.

Untreated hemorrhoids can also make it difficult to control bowel movements. This can lead to fecal incontinence, which is when you are not able to control when you have a bowel movement. This can be extremely embarrassing and can make it difficult to live a normal life.

If you are experiencing any of these problems, it is important to see a doctor. Hemorrhoids can be a painful and embarrassing condition, but there are treatments available that can help.

Hemorrhoids are a common problem that can be painful and uncomfortable. However, there are many ways to treat them, and most people can find relief. If you are suffering from hemorrhoids, talk to your doctor about the best treatment options for you.

When should I go to the doctor for external hemorrhoids?

External hemorrhoids can be painful and itchy, and can sometimes bleed. They happen when blood vessels in the anal or rectal area become larger and engorged. This can happen for a variety of reasons, including straining during a bowel movement, pregnancy, or sitting for long periods of time on the toilet.

If you have external hemorrhoids, you may notice that they feel like lumps near your anus. They may be itchy, and you may see blood on toilet paper or in the toilet bowl after a bowel movement. In some cases, external hemorrhoids can be so large that they protrude from the anus.

If you have any of these symptoms, you should see your doctor. They can confirm that you have hemorrhoids and recommend treatment. Treatment for external hemorrhoids may include cream or ointments to reduce inflammation, stool softeners to reduce straining, and over-the-counter pain relief. In some cases, surgery may be necessary to remove the hemorrhoids.

If you are experiencing pain, bleeding, or itching from your hemorrhoids, make an appointment to see your doctor. They will be able to recommend the best treatment for you.

Do external hemorrhoids always burst?

There are two main types of hemorrhoids: internal and external. Internal hemorrhoids are located inside the rectum, and therefore are not visible. External hemorrhoids are located under the skin around the anus, and can be seen and felt.

Hemorrhoids are often caused by straining during a bowel movement, pregnancy, or obesity. They can also be caused by sitting for long periods of time on the toilet.

External hemorrhoids can sometimes burst. This usually happens when the hemorrhoid becomes too full of blood and the surrounding tissue can no longer contain it. When this happens, the blood will leak out of the hemorrhoid and can cause severe pain.

If an external hemorrhoid does burst, it is important to clean the area with warm water and soap. If the bleeding is severe, it is important to seek medical attention.

If you are suffering from hemorrhoids, you are not alone. Hemorrhoids are a very common condition that affects people of all ages. There are a number of treatments available that can help to relieve the symptoms of hemorrhoids. If home treatment does not work, or if the hemorrhoids are severe, you may need to see a doctor.

Why do you get external hemorrhoids?

External hemorrhoids occur when the anal veins become dilated or enlarge. This happens when there is increased pressure on these veins, often from straining during a bowel movement. The added pressure causes the veins to bulge and swell. External hemorrhoids can be very painful if the area becomes irritated or damaged.

There are a number of things that can contribute to the development of external hemorrhoids. One of the most common is chronic constipation. When people are constipated, they often strain excessively during bowel movements. This puts added pressure on the anal veins and can cause them to become dilated over time.

Pregnancy is another common cause of external hemorrhoids. This is due to the increased pressure on the anal veins that occurs during pregnancy. Hemorrhoids are also more common in people who are overweight or obese. This is because there is added pressure on the anal veins when carrying extra weight.

If you are suffering from external hemorrhoids, there are a number of things you can do to get relief. One of the most effective treatments is to soak the area in warm water. This can help to soothe the pain and irritation. You can also try using a hemorrhoid cream or ointment. These can help to reduce swelling and inflammation. If your hemorrhoids are severe, you may need to see a doctor for treatment.

Hemorrhoids are a common and uncomfortable problem that can be effectively treated with lifestyle changes and medical interventions. With proper care, most people with hemorrhoids can experience relief from their symptoms.

Can exercise help hemorrhoids?

Hemorrhoids are very common—nearly 75% of Americans will have them at some point in their lives. They're often painful and can make everyday activities, like sitting or going to the bathroom, extremely uncomfortable. Many people turn to over-the-counter treatments or home remedies to ease the symptoms of hemorrhoids. But can exercise also be helpful?

The short answer is yes, exercising can help hemorrhoids in a few ways. First, when you exercise, you help maintain a healthy weight. Being overweight puts extra pressure on your pelvis and can make hemorrhoids worse. Exercise also helps to relieve constipation, which is a common cause of hemorrhoids. Constipation happens when your stool is hard and dry, making it difficult to pass. This can cause the veins in your anus or rectum to become swollen and painful.

There are a few specific exercises that can help hemorrhoids, too. Kegel exercises, for example, can help to strengthen your pelvic floor muscles. This can improve your bowel movements and reduce the pressure on your hemorrhoids. Yoga poses like Child's Pose and Cobra Pose can also help to ease constipation and relieve pressure on your hemorrhoids.

Of course, if you're experiencing pain from hemorrhoids, you'll want to avoid anything that puts extra pressure on that area. That means no straining or lifting heavy weights. If you're just starting to exercise, be sure to listen to your body and take things slowly at first.

If you're struggling with hemorrhoids, adding some exercise to your routine may be just what you need to find relief.

Can exercise help prevent me from getting hemorrhoids?

Hemorrhoids are often the result of constipation and straining during bowel movements. Exercise can help to prevent constipation by keeping the bowels regular. Regular exercise can also help to reduce the amount of straining required during bowel movements.

There are a number of different exercises that can help to prevent constipation and reduce the risk of developing hemorrhoids. Some examples of exercises that can help include: walking, jogging, swimming, and biking. These exercises can help to increase the muscle tone in the abdominal and pelvic areas, which can help to reduce the strain on the bowel during movements.

Additionally, there are a number of specific exercises that can help to target the muscles in the pelvic area. These exercises can help to reduce the risk of straining during bowel movements and can also help to prevent the development of hemorrhoids. Some examples of these specific exercises include: Kegel exercises, planks, and bridges.

Overall, exercise can be a helpful tool in preventing constipation and the development of hemorrhoids. However, it is important to consult with a doctor before beginning any new exercise regimen, particularly if you are over the age of 50 or if you have any other health concerns.

What is the best exercise to get rid of hemorrhoids?

It is common for people to ask what the best exercise is to get rid of hemorrhoids. Unfortunately, there is no one definitive answer to this question. The best exercise for hemorrhoids may vary depending on the individual and the severity of their condition.

For those who are suffering from mild hemorrhoids, simple lifestyle changes may be all that is needed in order to provide relief. This includes things like eating a high-fiber diet, drinking plenty of water, and getting regular exercise. These lifestyle changes can help to promote regular bowel movements and reduce the strain on the anal area.

Those who are suffering from more severe hemorrhoids may need to take things a step further in order to find relief. One option is to try a specific exercise routine designed to improve circulation and reduce strain on the anal area. Another option is to use a hemorrhoid cream or ointment, which can help to soothe the area and provide some relief from symptoms.

If lifestyle changes and home remedies are not providing enough relief, it is important to consult with a doctor. They will be able to provide more specific advice on the best exercise for hemorrhoids based on the individual's situation. In some cases, surgery may be necessary in order to remove the hemorrhoids.

There is no one definitive answer to the question of what the best exercise is to get rid of hemorrhoids. The best course of action may vary depending on the individual and the severity of their condition. It is important to consult with a doctor if lifestyle changes and home remedies are not providing enough relief.

Discussions about hemorrhoids are oftentimes uncomfortable, but they are nothing to be embarrassed about. This common condition affects millions of Americans every year. Hemorrhoids can be mild or severe, temporary or permanent. There are many different treatment options available, so it is important to speak with a doctor to determine the best course of action. With proper treatment, hemorrhoids can be managed and even cured.

At what age do people start getting hemorrhoids?

Hemorrhoids are swollen blood vessels in the anal or rectal area. They can be internal, which means they're inside the rectum. Or they can be external, which means they're outside the anus. Most people have hemorrhoids at some point in their lives.

Hemorrhoids develop when there's extra pressure on the anal or rectal veins. This can happen during pregnancy, when you're constipated, or when you sit on the toilet for long periods of time. The pressure causes the veins to swell and makes them painful.

If you have hemorrhoids, you may experience bleeding during a bowel movement, itching, or pain. You may also see blood on toilet paper or in the toilet bowl.

Hemorrhoids are more likely to develop as you age. That's because the supporting tissues around the anal and rectal veins weaken as you get older.

There are a number of things you can do to prevent hemorrhoids, such as:

-eating a high-fiber diet

-avoiding constipation

-avoiding sitting on the toilet for long periods of time

-exercising regularly

If you do develop hemorrhoids, there are a number of treatments that can help, including:

-over-the-counter creams and ointments

-prescription creams and ointments

-sitz baths

-surgery

If you're experiencing hemorrhoids, you're not alone. Hemorrhoids are a common condition that can cause bleeding, pain, itching, and discomfort. There are a number of different treatments available, and the best treatment for you will depend on the severity of your symptoms. Be sure to talk to your doctor about your options so that you can find the best treatment for you.

How common are hemorrhoids?

Hemorrhoids are one of the most common medical conditions. They are caused by enlarged veins in the lower rectum and anus. Hemorrhoids can be internal (inside the rectum) or external (under the skin around the anus).

Most people with hemorrhoids will have no symptoms. Others may have itching, burning, and pain around the anus. If the hemorrhoids are large, they may cause bleeding during a bowel movement.

Hemorrhoids are most common in people between the ages of 45 and 65. They are also more common in women than in men.

There are a number of things that can increase your risk of developing hemorrhoids. These include:

- Constipation or diarrhea

- Straining during bowel movements

- Pregnancy

- Anal intercourse

- Obesity

- A sedentary lifestyle

If you have hemorrhoids, there are a number of things you can do to relieve your symptoms. These include:

- Taking over-the-counter pain relievers such as acetaminophen or ibuprofen

- Applying over-the-counter hemorrhoid creams or ointments

- Taking warm baths

- avoiding sitting for long periods of time

If your symptoms are severe or persistent, you may need to see a doctor. Treatment options include:

- Rubber band ligation, in which a rubber band is placed around the base of the hemorrhoid to cut off its blood supply.

- Sclerotherapy, in which a chemical solution is injected into the hemorrhoid to shrink it.

- Hemorrhoidectomy, in which the hemorrhoid is surgically removed.

Hemorrhoids are a very common condition, affecting millions of people worldwide. While they can be painful and uncomfortable, most cases can be treated at home with over-the-counter medications. In severe cases, surgery may be necessary.

Hemorrhoids are an extremely common condition, affecting millions of people worldwide. Although they can be painful and uncomfortable, they are usually not serious. With proper treatment, most hemorrhoids will go away within a few days. There are a number of effective treatments available, so if you are suffering from hemorrhoids, be sure to talk to your doctor to find the best option for you.

Do teens get hemorrhoids?

Hemorrhoids are a common problem for people of all ages, but they can be especially difficult for teens. The problem is that hemorrhoids can be very painful and can make it hard to sit or stand for long periods of time. If you are a teenager and you think you may have hemorrhoids, it is important to see a doctor for a proper diagnosis.

There are two types of hemorrhoids: internal and external. Internal hemorrhoids are located inside the rectum and are usually not painful. External hemorrhoids are located under the skin around the anus and can be very painful. Hemorrhoids are usually caused by straining during a bowel movement, pregnancy, or obesity.

If you have hemorrhoids, there are several things you can do to ease the pain and discomfort. For example, you can try over-the-counter creams or ointments, use a hemorrhoidal cream or ointment, or take a sitz bath. You should also avoid straining during a bowel movement and eat a high-fiber diet to avoid constipation. If home treatment doesn't work, you may need to see a doctor for a more serious treatment.

If you suffer from hemorrhoids, you're not alone. Millions of Americans suffer from this often embarrassing and painful condition. But there are things you can do to get relief. Talk to your doctor about the best treatment options for you, and make sure to follow his or her advice. With proper treatment, most hemorrhoids can be managed successfully.

Chapter Seventeen

Do children get hemorrhoids?

Hemorrhoids are a common condition, affecting both men and women of all ages. In most cases, they are not serious and can be treated at home with over-the-counter medications. However, in some cases, hemorrhoids can become more severe, leading to surgery.

So, do children get hemorrhoids? The answer is yes, children can get hemorrhoids, although it is more common in adults. Hemorrhoids are caused by a variety of things, including constipation, sitting on the toilet for a long time, pregnancy, and obesity. Treatment for hemorrhoids in children is typically the same as for adults, and includes over-the-counter creams and ointments, sitz baths, and increased fiber in the diet. In some cases, hemorrhoids may go away on their own without treatment. However, if hemorrhoids are severe or do not go away, surgery may be necessary.

What herbal can cure hemorrhoids?

There are many different herbs that can potentially cure hemorrhoids. Some of the most popular and effective herbs include Aloe vera, which is known for its healing properties, and Witch hazel, which can help to soothe and heal the affected area. Other popular herbs include garlic, which has natural antibiotic properties, and ginger, which can help to reduce inflammation.

What home remedy shrinks hemorrhoids fast?

There are a number of different home remedies that can shrink hemorrhoids fast. One popular method is to sit in a warm bath for fifteen minutes a day. This dilates the blood vessels and helps to reduce inflammation.

Another effective home remedy is to apply a cold compress to the area for fifteen minutes a day. This helps to shrink the swollen blood vessels and reduce pain and inflammation.

Witch hazel is a natural astringent that can also be very effective in shrinking hemorrhoids. Apply Witch hazel to a cotton ball and place it on the area for fifteen minutes. This will help to soothe and shrink the swollen vessels.

Aloe vera gel is also a very effective home remedy for hemorrhoids. Apply the gel directly to the area and allow it to sit for fifteen minutes. This will help to reduce inflammation and pain.

There are a number of different home remedies that can help to shrink hemorrhoids fast. Try a few and see which one works best for you.

Is there a natural way to remove hemorrhoids?

Hemorrhoids are a painful and potentially embarrassing condition that can happen to anyone. They are caused by the swelling of veins in the anal or rectal area, and can make everyday activities like sitting or going to the bathroom incredibly uncomfortable.

There are a number of things that can cause hemorrhoids, including constipation, sitting for long periods of time, and pregnancy. Fortunately, there are also a number of things you can do to get rid of hemorrhoids or prevent them from happening in the first place.

One of the most effective ways to get rid of hemorrhoids is to increase your fiber intake. This can be done by eating more high-fiber foods like fruits, vegetables, and whole grains, or by taking a fiber supplement. Fiber will help to soften your stools, making them easier to pass and less likely to irritate your hemorrhoids.

Another helpful tip is to avoid sitting or standing for long periods of time. If your job requires you to sit or stand for long periods, take frequent breaks to walk around and stretch your legs. Also, when going to the bathroom, try to avoid straining or holding your breath, as this can also aggravate hemorrhoids.

If you are already dealing with hemorrhoids, there are a number of over-the-counter treatments that can help to relieve your symptoms. These include creams, ointments, and suppositories that can be applied topically to the affected area. You can also take a sitz bath, which is a special type of bath that allows you to soak the affected area in warm water for relief.

In some cases, hemorrhoids may require more aggressive treatment. If home remedies and over-the-counter treatments are not providing relief, your doctor may recommend a procedure to remove the hemorrhoids. Surgery is generally only recommended for severe cases that have not responded to other treatments.

If you are concerned about hemorrhoids, talk to your doctor. They can help to determine the cause of your hemorrhoids and recommend the best course of treatment. With the right approach, hemorrhoids can be managed effectively and with minimal discomfort.

What shrinks hemorrhoids fast?

There are a number of things that can help shrink hemorrhoids fast. These include:

- Soaking the affected area in warm water for 15 minutes several times a day. This can helps to reduce inflammation and pain.

- Applying a cold compress to the area for a few minutes at a time. This can also help to reduce swelling.

- Taking over-the-counter medications such as ibuprofen or acetaminophen to help reduce pain.

- Applying topical ointments or creams to the area. This can help to soothe the skin and reduce irritation.

- Avoiding constipation by eating a high-fiber diet and drinking plenty of fluids. This can help to reduce strain during bowel movements and prevent further irritation of the hemorrhoids.

- Avoiding sitting or standing for long periods of time. This can help to reduce pressure on the hemorrhoids.

- Wearing loose, comfortable clothing. This can help to reduce irritation and chafing.

following these tips can help to shrink hemorrhoids fast and provide relief from discomfort.

What to drink to heal hemorrhoids?

If you're suffering from hemorrhoids, you're probably wondering what you can do to get relief. You may be surprised to learn that one of the best things you can do is to drink lots of fluids. That's because staying hydrated helps to keep your stool soft, which makes it easier to pass. It also helps to reduce inflammation and irritation.

So what fluids should you drink? Water is always a good choice, but you can also try juices or herbal teas. Just avoid caffeine and alcohol, which can dehydrate you. You might also want to try a stool softener like Miralax, which can be mixed into any beverage.

If you're struggling to get enough fluids, try carrying around a water bottle with you so you can take sips throughout the day. You might also want to eat foods that are high in water content, such as fruits and vegetables. And finally, if you're having trouble going to the bathroom, don't be afraid to ask your doctor about a laxative.

Hemorrhoids can be a real pain in the you-know-what. But don't fret, there are plenty of things you can do to get rid of them. From home remedies to over-the-counter treatments, there's something out there that will work for you. So, don't be afraid to ask for help if you're having a hard time dealing with your hemorrhoids.

What herbal can cure hemorrhoids?

There are many different herbs that have been traditionally used to treat hemorrhoids. Some of the most popular include aloe vera, witch hazel, and gotu kola.

Aloe vera has been used for centuries to treat a variety of ailments, and hemorrhoids are no exception. This plant is thought to be effective in relieving pain, inflammation, and itching associated with hemorrhoids.

Witch hazel is another popular herbal remedy for hemorrhoids. This plant extract is thought to be effective in reducing inflammation and swelling. It can be applied topically to the affected area.

Gotu kola is an herb that is sometimes used to treat hemorrhoids. This plant is thought to be effective in reducing inflammation, pain, and itching. It can be taken orally or applied topically to the affected area.

What home remedy shrinks hemorrhoids fast?

Hemorrhoids are one of the most common medical conditions in the world, affecting millions of people each year. While there are many over-the-counter and prescription medications available to treat hemorrhoids, there are also several home remedies that can shrink hemorrhoids fast.

One of the most effective home remedies for hemorrhoids is to increase your intake of dietary fiber. Fiber helps to soften stool and make it easier to pass, which can reduce the pain and bleeding associated with hemorrhoids. Foods that are high in fiber include fruits, vegetables, whole grains, and beans. You should aim to consume 25-38 grams of fiber each day.

If you are constipated, this can also worsen hemorrhoids. To help relieve constipation, drink plenty of fluids and eat foods that are high in water content, such as soup, broth, or watery fruits and vegetables. You can also take a stool softener or laxative if needed.

Sitting for long periods of time can also make hemorrhoids worse, so try to stand up and move around every few hours. If you must sit for an extended period, take a break every 20 minutes or so to stand up and walk around. And when you do sit, be sure to use a donut-shaped pillow to relieve pressure on the area.

Applying ice to the area can also help to reduce pain and swelling. Simply wrap an ice pack in a towel and apply it to the affected area for 10-15 minutes at a time.

Finally, there are several over-the-counter hemorrhoid creams and ointments that can provide relief from symptoms. Be sure to read the labels carefully and follow the directions for use.

Is there a natural way to remove hemorrhoids?

Hemorrhoids are swollen blood vessels in and around the anus and lower rectum. They are a common and often painful problem. Many people seek out natural ways to remove hemorrhoids. Here are a few things you can try.

Diet: Eating a high-fiber diet is one of the best ways to soften stools, which reduces the pressure on hemorrhoids. A fiber-rich diet includes foods like beans, whole grains, and leafy greens.

Exercise: Regular exercise can help reduce the risk of constipation and strain during bowel movements.

Hygiene: Keeping the anal area clean is important. Wiping carefully and using moist wipes or cotton balls dipped in warm water can help.

Sitz baths: Soaking the anal area in a sitz bath can help reduce swelling and pain.

topically applied creams and ointments: Many topical treatments are available over the counter to help with the symptoms of hemorrhoids.

There are many natural ways to remove hemorrhoids. Some people find that making lifestyle changes, such as diet and exercise, helps to reduce hemorrhoids. Others find relief with home remedies, such as sitz baths and topical treatments.

What shrinks hemorrhoids fast?

There is nothing worse than the itching, burning, and pain that hemorrhoids can cause. If you are looking for a fast and effective way to shrink your hemorrhoids, you have come to the right place.

There are a few things you can do to shrink your hemorrhoids fast. First, you can try using a hemorrhoid cream or ointment. These creams and ointments will help to soothe your hemorrhoids and make them feel better. Second, you can take a sitz bath. A sitz bath is a warm bath that you can take to help relieve the pain and itchiness of hemorrhoids. Third, you can try using a cold compress. A cold compress will help to shrink your hemorrhoids and make them feel less inflamed. Fourth, you can try using a stool softener. A stool softener will help to make your stool less hard, which will make it easier to pass and will help to reduce the pain and inflammation of hemorrhoids. Fifth, you can try increasing your fiber intake. Fiber will help to make your stool softer and will also help to reduce the pain and inflammation of hemorrhoids.

There are a few things that you should avoid if you want to shrink your hemorrhoids fast. First, you should avoid straining during bowel movements. Straining can aggravate your hemorrhoids and make them worse. Second, you should avoid sitting for long periods of time. Sitting for long periods of time can aggravate your hemorrhoids and make them worse. Third, you should avoid sitting on hard surfaces. Sitting on hard surfaces can aggravate your hemorrhoids and make them worse. Fourth, you should avoid rubbing your hemorrhoids. Rubbing your hemorrhoids can aggravate your hemorrhoids and make them worse.

If you follow these tips, you should be able to shrink your hemorrhoids fast. If you find that your hemorrhoids are still not shrinking, you may want to consider seeing a doctor to find out if you need to have surgery to remove them.

What to drink to heal hemorrhoids?

There are many different things that people can do in order to help heal their hemorrhoids. This can include changing their diet, taking certain medications, or even surgery. However, one thing that people may not think about is what they drink. There are actually certain drinks that can help heal hemorrhoids.

One of the best things that people can drink is water. This is because water can help to keep the body hydrated, which is important when healing any wound. It is also important to avoid caffeine and alcohol, as these can act as diuretics and cause dehydration.

Another good drink to help heal hemorrhoids is fresh vegetable juice. This is because it can help to reduce inflammation and provide the body with nutrients that it needs to heal. Fresh fruit juices can also be beneficial, but it is important to avoid those with high sugar content as this can actually make hemorrhoids worse.

There are also a few teas that can be helpful in healing hemorrhoids. Some good options include chamomile tea, witch hazel tea, and lavender tea. These teas can help to soothe the skin and reduce inflammation.

Finally, it is also important to make sure that you are getting enough fiber in your diet. This is because fiber can help to soften stool and make it easier to pass. This can be found in whole grains, fruits, and vegetables.

How common are hemorrhoids?

Hemorrhoids are one of the most common medical conditions. It is estimated that 50% of the world population has hemorrhoids by the time they reach the age of 50. In the United States, it is estimated that 10 million people have hemorrhoids.

Hemorrhoids are more common in developed countries, such as the United States. This is likely due to the higher level of stress and the Western diet, which is low in fiber.

There are two types of hemorrhoids, internal and external. Internal hemorrhoids are usually not painful, but can bleed. External hemorrhoids are usually painful and can bleed.

Hemorrhoids are usually not serious, but can be painful and uncomfortable. If you have hemorrhoids, there are several things you can do to relieve the symptoms. These include:

- Taking over-the-counter pain relievers, such as ibuprofen or acetaminophen

- Applying a hemorrhoid cream or ointment to the affected area

- Taking a sitz bath (a bath in which you sit in warm water for a short period of time)

- Using moist toilet paper or wipes

- Avoiding constipation by eating a high-fiber diet and drinking plenty of fluids

If home treatment does not work, you may need to see a doctor. The doctor can prescribe stronger pain relievers or recommend other treatments, such as a bulkectomy (removal of the hemorrhoid) or rubber band ligation (a procedure to tie off the hemorrhoid).

If you have hemorrhoids, you are not alone. Many people have hemorrhoids, and there are a number of effective treatments available. The best way to treat hemorrhoids is to avoid them in the first place. To do this, you can eat a high-fiber diet, drink plenty of fluids, and exercise regularly. If you do develop hemorrhoids, there are a number of effective treatment options available, so you do not need to suffer.

What actually shrinks hemorrhoids?

Hemorrhoids are swollen blood vessels in the lower rectum or anus. They can be painful and sometimes bleed. Hemorrhoids are common, affecting up to 25% of adults in the United States.

There are different types of hemorrhoids, and each type has its own set of causes and symptoms. Internal hemorrhoids are located inside the anus or rectum, while external hemorrhoids are found under the skin around the anus.

Hemorrhoids are usually caused by increased pressure in the lower rectum or anus. This can happen for a number of reasons, including pregnancy, constipation, or straining during bowel movements.

There are a number of treatment options for hemorrhoids, and the best option for you will depends on the severity of your symptoms. For milder cases, over-the-counter creams and ointments can be effective in reducing pain and inflammation.

If you have more severe symptoms, your doctor may recommend a more aggressive treatment, such as a hemorrhoidectomy, which is a surgery to remove the hemorrhoids. There are also a number of nonsurgical treatments that can be effective, such as sclerotherapy, which is a procedure that injects a chemical solution into the hemorrhoids to shrink them.

In most cases, hemorrhoids can be treated at home with over-the-counter products and lifestyle changes, such as drinking more fluids, eating a high-fiber diet, and avoiding constipation. However, if your symptoms are severe or persist, it's important to see your doctor to rule out other potential causes and get the appropriate treatment.

What not to do with hemorrhoids?

Hemorrhoids are a common and uncomfortable problem that can be tricky to treat. While there are many different ways to get rid of hemorrhoids, there are also a few things that you should avoid doing. Here are a few things not to do if you have hemorrhoids.

First, resist the urge to scratch. It may be tempting to scratch an itch, but this can actually make hemorrhoids worse. Scratching can cause the hemorrhoids to bleed and become more irritated.

Second, don't sit for long periods of time. This can put pressure on the hemorrhoids and make them worse. If you must sit for a long time, try to get up and move around every few hours.

Third, don't strain when you go to the bathroom. This can also make hemorrhoids worse. If you're having trouble going to the bathroom, try drinking plenty of fluids and eating high-fiber foods to help make things easier.

Fourth, don't use over-the-counter hemorrhoid treatments for more than a week. If your symptoms don't improve after a week of treatment, see your doctor.

Finally, avoid Foods that are difficult to digest can make hemorrhoids worse. So, if you have hemorrhoids, you might want to avoid foods like spicy foods, cheese, and caffeine.

How long should it take to shrink a hemorrhoid?

It is estimated that over half of the world's population will experience hemorrhoids at some point in their lives. So, how long should it take to shrink a hemorrhoid?

There are two main types of hemorrhoids: internal and external. Internal hemorrhoids are found inside the rectum and are usually not painful. External hemorrhoids are found under the skin around the anus and can be very painful.

Most hemorrhoids can be treated at home with over-the-counter (OTC) creams and ointments, stool softeners, warm baths, and ice packs. Some people may need to see a doctor for prescription-strength medication or surgery.

It can take anywhere from a few days to a couple of weeks for a hemorrhoid to shrink. The specific timeline depends on the type of hemorrhoid, the severity, and the treatment.

If you have an external hemorrhoid, you may feel a hard lump near your anus. This is called a thrombosed hemorrhoid and is usually very painful. If a blood clot forms in the hemorrhoid, it will need to be removed by a doctor. This usually requires a minor surgery.

After a thrombosed hemorrhoid is removed, the swelling and pain should go down within a week or so. If you have an internal hemorrhoid, it may take a bit longer for it to shrink. This is because the blood vessels inside the rectum are much larger than those in the anus.

If your hemorrhoids are severe, you may need to see a doctor for treatment. This is especially true if you're having difficulty going to the bathroom, your hemorrhoids are bleeding, or you're in a lot of pain.

There are a few different options for treating hemorrhoids. Your doctor may recommend a cream or ointment to help reduce the swelling. If the hemorrhoids are very large, you may need to have them surgically removed.

In most cases, hemorrhoids will go away on their own within a few days to a couple of weeks. However, if you have severe hemorrhoids, you may need to see a doctor for treatment.

If you think you have hemorrhoids, the first step is to see a doctor for a proper diagnosis. Many people have hemorrhoids, but have no symptoms. If you have hemorrhoids, there are a number of treatments that can help, depending on the severity of your symptoms. These include over-the-counter creams and suppositories, dietary changes, and home remedies. In some cases, surgery may be necessary.

Why won't my hemorrhoids shrink?

There are many reasons why your hemorrhoids may not be shrinking. If you're not sure what's causing your hemorrhoids, talk to your doctor. Here are some possible causes of why your hemorrhoids are not shrinking:

1. You're not using the right topical treatment - If you're not using the right topical treatment, your hemorrhoids may not shrink. Be sure to talk to your doctor about what topical treatments are best for you.

2. You're not using enough treatment - If you're only using a small amount of topical treatment, it may not be enough to shrink your hemorrhoids. Be sure to talk to your doctor about how much treatment you should be using.

3. You're not using the treatment often enough - If you're only using the topical treatment once or twice a day, it may not be enough to shrink your

hemorrhoids. Be sure to talk to your doctor about how often you should be using the treatment.

4. You're not using the right oral medication - If you're taking an oral medication for your hemorrhoids, but it's not the right one, it could be why your hemorrhoids are not shrinking. Be sure to talk to your doctor about what oral medication is best for you.

5. You're not following a high-fiber diet - A high-fiber diet is essential for shrinking hemorrhoids. Be sure to eat plenty of high-fiber foods, such as fruits, vegetables, and whole grains.

6. You're not drinking enough fluids - Drinking plenty of fluids is essential for shrinking hemorrhoids. Be sure to drink at least eight glasses of water a day.

7. You're not getting enough exercise - Exercise is essential for shrinking hemorrhoids. Be sure to get at least 30 minutes of exercise a day.

8. You're smoking - Smoking can make hemorrhoids worse. If you smoke, it's important to quit.

9. You're drinking too much alcohol - Drinking too much alcohol can make hemorrhoids worse. If you drink alcohol, it's important to drink in moderation.

10. You have a medical condition that's causing your hemorrhoids - There are a number of medical conditions that can cause hemorrhoids. If you have a medical condition, such as obesity, heart disease, or constipation, it's important to talk to your doctor about how to treat it.

How long does it take for a hemorrhoid to go away?

There is no one-size-fits-all answer to this question, as the duration of time it takes for a hemorrhoid to improve can vary depending on the individual case. However, there are some general guidelines that can provide some insight.

For instance, hemorrhoids that are caused by pregnancy or childbirth generally improve within a few weeks after the baby is delivered. Other cases may improve with home treatment, such as increase fiber in the diet, stool softeners, and over-the-counter creams. In more severe cases, hemorrhoids may require surgery.

In general, the prognosis for hemorrhoids is good, and most people experience relief from symptoms within a few days to weeks. However, it is important to followup with a healthcare provider to ensure that the hemorrhoids are properly treated to avoid complications.

What drinks make hemorrhoids worse?

Hemorrhoids are often thought of as a minor problem, but they can cause a great deal of discomfort. There are a number of things that can make hemorrhoids worse, and one of them is the type of drinks you consume.

Certain drinks can act as diuretics, which means they promote urination. This can lead to dehydration, and that can in turn make hemorrhoids worse. Caffeinated beverages are some of the worst offenders in this regard. Coffee, tea, soda, and even chocolate can all act as diuretics. Alcohol is another type of drink that can promote urination, so it's best to avoid that if you're trying to relieve hemorrhoids.

Drinks that are high in sugar can also contribute to hemorrhoids. Sugar can cause inflammation in the body, and that can make hemorrhoids worse. Fruit juices, sports drinks, and even some types of milk are all high in sugar.

You're better off sticking to water or unsweetened beverages if you want to avoid making your hemorrhoids worse.

Of course, you don't have to give up all of your favorite drinks if you have hemorrhoids. Just be mindful of what you're drinking, and try to avoid the beverages that are most likely to make your symptoms worse.

What drinks to avoid with hemorrhoids?

When you have hemorrhoids, there are certain drinks you should avoid. Drinks that can irritate your stomach or cause you to become constipated can make your hemorrhoids worse.

Some of the worst offenders are alcoholic beverages. Alcohol can dehydrate you, and when you're dehydrated, your body doesn't function as well. This can lead to constipation, which can worsen hemorrhoids. Alcohol can also irritate your stomach, which can also make hemorrhoids worse.

Coffee and other caffeinated beverages can also be problematic. Caffeine is a diuretic, so it can lead to dehydration. Dehydration can cause constipation, which can make hemorrhoids worse. Caffeine can also irritate your stomach, which can make hemorrhoids worse.

Carbonated beverages can also be problematic. Carbonation can cause bloating, which can put pressure on your hemorrhoids and make them worse. Carbonated beverages can also irritate your stomach, which can make hemorrhoids worse.

It's best to avoid any beverages that might dehydrate you, irritate your stomach, or cause you to become constipated. This includes alcoholic beverages, caffeinated beverages, and carbonated beverages. Drink plenty of water and other fluids that will keep you hydrated and help you avoid becoming constipated.

If you're suffering from hemorrhoids, you're not alone. Hemorrhoids are a common ailment, especially among pregnant women and those who are constipated. There are a number of treatments available, both over-the-counter and through your doctor. With proper treatment and self-care, your hemorrhoids will soon be a thing of the past.

Can I use a pin to pop my hemorrhoids?

It's a common question people ask when they discover they have hemorrhoids – can I just pop them like a pimple? Unfortunately, the answer is no. Popping hemorrhoids can cause them to rupture and bleed, which can lead to additional pain and discomfort. It can also cause the hemorrhoids to become more inflamed and irritated. If you must pop a hemorrhoid, it's best to do it with a sterile needle or other sharp object that won't tear the tissue.

Does it hurt to pop a hemorrhoid?

Most everyone has had hemorrhoids at one time or another. They occur when veins in the anus and rectum become swollen and inflamed. Hemorrhoids can be internal, occurring inside the rectum, or external, developing under the skin around the anus.

There are a number of different ways to treat hemorrhoids, but one of the most common is to simply pop them. This may seem counterintuitive, but popping a hemorrhoid can actually help to reduce the inflammation and pain associated with the condition.

Of course, as with any medical procedure, there are some risks involved with popping a hemorrhoid. The most common complication is that the hemorrhoid may bleed. This usually isn't serious and will resolve on its own, but it can be unsettling.

Another potential complication is that the hemorrhoid may become infected. This is more likely to happen if the skin around the anus is already irritated or broken. If you notice that the area around your popped hemorrhoid is red, swollen, or oozing pus, you should see a doctor right away.

Overall, popping a hemorrhoid is generally safe and can be an effective way to find relief from the discomfort. Just be sure to consult with a doctor first to make sure that your hemorrhoids are ready to be popped.

Overall, hemorrhoids are a painful condition that can be difficult to manage. However, there are treatments available that can help to provide relief. It is important to speak with a doctor if hemorrhoids are causing discomfort, as they can determine the best course of treatment.

What not to do with hemorrhoids?

There aren't a whole lot of things you can do wrong when it comes to hemorrhoids, but there are a few. Here are some things you should avoid doing if you have hemorrhoids.

First and foremost, don't scratch. It might feel tempting, but trust us, it's not worth it. Scratching will only make the itching worse and could lead to further irritation and even bleeding.

Second, don't sit for long periods of time. This can put unnecessary pressure on the hemorrhoids and make them swell even more. Try to take breaks often and move around as much as possible.

Third, don't strain when you go to the bathroom. This can again lead to more pressure on the hemorrhoids and make them bleed. Instead, try to relax and let everything come out naturally.

Lastly, don't try any home remedies that you find online without first consulting your doctor. Some of these home remedies can actually make the hemorrhoids worse.

So there you have it, a few things to avoid doing if you have hemorrhoids. by following these simple tips, you can help reduce the pain and irritation caused by hemorrhoids.

If you have hemorrhoids, you're not alone. Hemorrhoids are common and usually not too serious. They can often be treated with home remedies, and you may not need to see a doctor. But some types of hemorrhoids can cause more serious problems. If your hemorrhoids are very painful or are bleeding, you should see your doctor.

should I pop my hemorrhoids?

A common question people suffering from hemorrhoids ask is whether or not they should pop their hemorrhoids. The answer to this question is usually a resounding “no” from healthcare professionals. This is because, while it may provide temporary relief, popping a hemorrhoid can often lead to further irritation and pain.

There are a number of reasons why you shouldn’t pop your hemorrhoids. For one, the act of popping a hemorrhoid can cause it to rupture and bleed. This can be extremely painful and may even lead to an infection. Additionally, when a hemorrhoid ruptures, it can cause the surrounding tissue to become inflamed, leading to further discomfort.

Additionally, popping a hemorrhoid can cause it to become thrombosed, meaning that a blood clot has formed within the hemorrhoid. This can be incredibly painful and can often require medical intervention to resolve.

So, while it may be tempting to pop your hemorrhoids in an attempt to find relief, it is generally not advised. If you are suffering from hemorrhoids, there are a number of other treatment options available that are much more effective and much less likely to cause further pain and irritation.

what happens if I pop my hemorrhoid?

Hemorrhoids are often painful and itchy. If you scratch or rub them, they can bleed. If you have a hemorrhoid that has prolapsed—meaning it has pushed through your anal opening—you may be able to see or feel it. And, it can be painful and uncomfortable.

If you have a prolapsed hemorrhoid, you may be tempted to push it back up. But, don't do this. It can be painful and make the hemorrhoid more likely to prolapse again.

If you have a hemorrhoid that is bleeding, you should see your doctor. Bleeding from a hemorrhoid is usually a sign that it is inflamed. In some cases, it can also be a sign of a more serious condition, such as colon cancer.

If you have a hemorrhoid that is causing pain or bleeding, your doctor may recommend surgery to remove it. Surgery is usually a last resort, and it is not always successful. In some cases, the hemorrhoid may come back.

There are many potential causes of hemorrhoids, including everything from genetics to constipation. However, there are also many treatments available, from simple self-care at home to surgery. If you're suffering from hemorrhoids, be sure to talk to your doctor to find the best course of treatment for you.

Are hemorrhoids more common when you get older?

Hemorrhoids are more common when you get older, but they can affect people of any age. The condition is usually the result of a build-up of pressure in the anal region, which can cause the veins in the area to become swollen and inflamed. Hemorrhoids can cause a great deal of discomfort, and can even lead to bleeding. In some cases, hemorrhoids can be cured with over-the-counter treatments or home remedies, but in other cases, surgery may be necessary.

If you're experiencing pain, bleeding, or itching in the anal area, you may have hemorrhoids. Although they can be embarrassing to talk about, hemorrhoids are actually a very common condition. While there is no cure for hemorrhoids, there are several things you can do to treat them and minimize your symptoms.

what are internal hemorrhoids?

Most people think of hemorrhoids as swollen, itchy veins in the anal region, but there is another type of hemorrhoid, called an internal hemorrhoid, which occurs higher up in the anal canal. Internal hemorrhoids are not visible from the outside, and often do not cause any discomfort. However, they can bleed, and sometimes prolapse, or bulge out, through the anal opening.

Internal hemorrhoids are classified into four grades, depending on their severity. Grade I hemorrhoids are small and swollen, but do not prolapse. Grade II hemorrhoids prolapse, but spontaneously return inside the anal canal. Grade III hemorrhoids prolapse and need to be manually pushed back in. Grade IV hemorrhoids are permanently prolapsed and cannot be pushed back in.

Symptoms of internal hemorrhoids can include bleeding during a bowel movement, mucus discharge, anal itchiness, and pain during a bowel movement. However, many people with internal hemorrhoids do not experience any symptoms.

Internal hemorrhoids are usually caused by increased pressure in the anal canal, which can be due to pregnancy, constipation, or diarrhea. Treatment for internal hemorrhoids depends on the grade and symptoms. For Grade I and II hemorrhoids, treatments can include increased fiber intake, stool softeners, and over-the-counter hemorrhoid creams or ointments. If these conservative measures do not improve symptoms, office-based procedures such as infrared coagulation or rubber band ligation can be done. Grade III and IV hemorrhoids may require surgical treatment.

what are external hemorrhoids?

External hemorrhoids are dilated blood vessels that form around the anal opening. They can be itchy and painful, and may bleed. Although they can be troubling, they are usually not serious.

There are a number of things that can cause or contribute to the formation of external hemorrhoids. One is straining during bowel movements. This can happen if you are constipated and have to strain to have a bowel movement, or if you have diarrhea and your stool is hard to pass. Pregnancy can also cause or contribute to the formation of external hemorrhoids, because the growing uterus puts pressure on the veins in the pelvis. Other causes include anal intercourse and sitting for long periods of time on the toilet.

External hemorrhoids can be treated a number of ways. If they are causing pain, witch hazel pads or cream can be applied to the area to help soothe. If they are itchy, a cream or ointment containing hydrocortisone can be helpful. If the hemorrhoids are large and painful, your doctor may recommend a hemorrhoidectomy, which is a surgical procedure to remove them.

In most cases, external hemorrhoids will go away on their own. But if they are causing you pain or discomfort, or if they bleed, talk to your doctor.

In conclusion, hemorrhoids are a common and often painful problem. Although they are not usually serious, they can be a nuisance. There are a number of things that you can do to ease the discomfort and pain of hemorrhoids. If home treatment does not work, or if the hemorrhoids are large and very painful, you may need to see a doctor.

What is a thrombosed hemorrhoid

A thrombosed hemorrhoid is a hemorrhoid that has developed a blood clot inside it. This can happen if the hemorrhoid becomes irritated or damaged. When this happens, the blood vessels inside the hemorrhoid can become inflamed and swollen. This can cause the hemorrhoid to bulge and prolapse, or protrude from the anus. If the blood clot forms inside the hemorrhoid, it is known as a thrombosed hemorrhoid.

Thrombosed hemorrhoids are typically painful. The pain is caused by the pressure of the blood clot inside the hemorrhoid. This pressure can cause the hemorrhoid to bulge and prolapse. It can also cause the blood vessels in the area to become inflamed and swollen. The pain is often worse when you sit down or stand up.

If you have a thrombosed hemorrhoid, you may notice that the area around the hemorrhoid is red and swollen. You may also see a blood clot in the area. The blood clot may be dark red or purple.

Thrombosed hemorrhoids usually occur in people who have a history of hemorrhoids. However, they can also occur in people who don't have a history of hemorrhoids.

There are a few things you can do to ease the pain of a thrombosed hemorrhoid. You can take a sitz bath, which is a warm bath that you take sitting in a few inches of water. You can also take over-the-counter pain medication, such as ibuprofen or acetaminophen. You can also apply a hemorrhoid cream or ointment to the area.

If the pain is severe, you may need to see a doctor. A doctor can prescribe stronger pain medication. If the thrombosed hemorrhoid is very large, the doctor may recommend surgery to remove it.

What happens if a thrombosed hemorrhoid pops?

If a thrombosed hemorrhoid pops, the individual may feel a sharp pain. This is because the blood clot that was causing the thrombosed hemorrhoid has now been released. In some cases, the individual may also see blood on toilet paper or in the toilet bowl.

It is important to seek medical attention if a thrombosed hemorrhoid pops. This is because the individual may be at risk for bleeding and infection. A medical professional will be able to properly clean the area and provide any necessary treatments.

If you are suffering from hemorrhoids, there are a few things you can do to get relief. These include over-the-counter medication, ointments, and creams. You can also try natural remedies such as witch hazel, aloe vera, or coconut oil. If you have severe hemorrhoids, you may need to see a doctor for treatment.

Can Epsom salt shrink hemorrhoids?

A common home treatment for hemorrhoids is to soak in a bath of warm water mixed with Epsom salt. Some people also find relief by applying a cold compress made with Epsom salt water to the affected area.

Epsom salt is a natural remedy that has been used for centuries to treat a variety of ailments. The salt is derived from mineral-rich waters in the Epsom area of Surrey, England.

Epsom salt is made up of magnesium sulfate, which is thought to be the active ingredient in the salt that provides the majority of its health benefits. Sulfates help improve the absorption of nutrients in the body and promote the elimination of toxins.

The magnesium in Epsom salt is also known for its anti-inflammatory properties. This means that it can help reduce swelling and inflammation in the tissues and vessels around the anus and lower rectum, which can contribute to the pain and discomfort associated with hemorrhoids.

While there is no scientific evidence to support the use of Epsom salt for hemorrhoids specifically, many people find that it provides relief from the symptoms associated with the condition. In addition, Epsom salt is a safe, natural remedy with few side effects.

It is estimated that over 50% of the population will suffer from hemorrhoids at some point in their lives. While hemorrhoids are usually not a serious condition, they can be very painful and uncomfortable. If you think you may have hemorrhoids, see your doctor for a diagnosis and treatment.

When Can a Hemorrhoid Pop?

A hemorrhoid is a swollen and inflamed blood vessel in the anal or rectal area. Hemorrhoids can occur inside the rectum (internal hemorrhoids), or they can occur under the skin around the anus (external hemorrhoids). Hemorrhoids are common, and they often occur after episodes of constipation or straining during a bowel movement.

Hemorrhoids are not usually painful, but they can cause bleeding during a bowel movement. Internal hemorrhoids may bleed into the toilet bowl, and external hemorrhoids may bleed into your underwear.

If a hemorrhoid becomes too large, it may prolapse, or pop out, through the anus. A prolapsed hemorrhoid can be very painful, and it can make bowel movements very difficult. If a hemorrhoid prolapses and cannot be pushed back into place, it will need to be treated by a doctor.

Hemorrhoids are often treated with over-the-counter creams or ointments, but more severe cases may require prescription medication or surgery.

There are many methods of treating hemorrhoids, from over-the-counter hemorrhoid creams to surgery. If you suspect that you have hemorrhoids, it is important to see your doctor to rule out other potential causes of your symptoms. If your hemorrhoids are mild, over-the-counter treatments may be all that you need. However, if your hemorrhoids are more severe, your doctor may recommend surgery. Hemorrhoids are a common condition, and there is no need to be embarrassed. Your doctor can help you find the treatment that is right for you.

What is a hemorrhoidectomy, and do I need one?

A hemorrhoidectomy is a surgical procedure to remove hemorrhoids. hemorrhoids are swollen and inflamed veins in the anal area.

There are two types of hemorrhoidectomies: a conventional hemorrhoidectomy and a stapled hemorrhoidectomy. In a conventional hemorrhoidectomy, the surgeon makes an incision in the anal area and removes the hemorrhoids. In a stapled hemorrhoidectomy, also called a hemorrhoidopexy, the surgeon uses a special device to staple and remove the hemorrhoids.

You may need a hemorrhoidectomy if you have severe hemorrhoids that don't respond to other treatments. You may also need a hemorrhoidectomy if you have hemorrhoids that are prolapsed, or bulging out, of your anus.

The surgery takes about 30 minutes. You will be given a local anesthetic to numb the area. You may also be given a sedative to help you relax.

After the surgery, you can expect to feel some pain and discomfort. Your doctor will prescribe pain medication and offer advice on how to manage the pain. You will also be given instructions on how to care for the area after surgery.

Most people recover from a hemorrhoidectomy within two to four weeks.

After reading this FAQ, you should have a better understanding of what hemorrhoids are and how to treat them. If you are experiencing any hemorrhoid symptoms, be sure to see a doctor to get proper treatment. With the right care, hemorrhoids can be managed and you can enjoy relief from your symptoms.

Why You Probably Don't Need Hemorrhoid Surgery

There are a lot of hemorrhoid treatments out there, but surgery isn't always the best option. In fact, surgery should be a last resort for treating hemorrhoids. Why? Because surgery is expensive, takes a long time to recover from, and doesn't always work.

Let's start with the cost of hemorrhoid surgery. The average cost of hemorrhoid surgery is $8,000. That's a lot of money! If you have health insurance, you will probably have to pay at least a part of this cost yourself.

Next, let's talk about recovery time. hemorrhoid surgery is a major surgery. You will be in the hospital for 3-5 days after the surgery. After you go home, you will need to take it easy for 2-4 weeks. This means no lifting, no straining, and no strenuous activity.

Finally, let's talk about the success rate of hemorrhoid surgery. The surgery has a high success rate, but that doesn't mean that it will work for everyone. Some people will still have hemorrhoids after the surgery.

So, if you are considering hemorrhoid surgery, think about the cost, the recovery time, and the success rate. Surgery should be a last resort for treating hemorrhoids.

There are many effective treatments for hemorrhoids, including over-the-counter preparations, prescription medications, and surgical options. With proper treatment, most people with hemorrhoids experience relief from symptoms and the hemorrhoids eventually go away.

What to Do if a Hemorrhoid Bursts

If a hemorrhoid bursts, it can be quite painful. There are a few things you can do to help ease the pain and heal the hemorrhoid.

First, try to clean the area with a soft cloth. This will help to remove any bacteria that could cause an infection. You can also use a hemorrhoid cream or ointment to help soothe the area.

If the pain is too much to bear, you can take a pain reliever such as ibuprofen. You should also drink plenty of fluids to help keep the area clean and to prevent dehydration.

If the hemorrhoid does not heal within a few days, or if it starts to bleed, you should see a doctor. They can prescribe a stronger cream or ointment, or they may recommend a procedure to remove the hemorrhoid.

Hemorrhoids are a common condition that can be painful and uncomfortable. Although they are not usually dangerous, they can be a nuisance. If you have hemorrhoids, there are several things you can do to relieve your symptoms. In most cases, simple lifestyle changes and home remedies are all you need to get relief.

How long does it take for a hemorrhoid to shrink completely?

It is difficult to provide an answer to the question of how long it will take for a hemorrhoid to completely shrink since there are a number of different factors that can influence this. The severity of the hemorrhoid, for example, will play a role in how long it takes to shrink. In general, however, it is possible for a hemorrhoid to take several weeks or even months to completely disappear.

There are a number of different methods that can be used in order to shrink a hemorrhoid. This can include over-the-counter creams and ointments, prescription medications, or even surgery in some cases. The method that is chosen will also play a role in how long it takes for the hemorrhoid to completely shrink.

In most cases, however, it is possible for a hemorrhoid to be effectively treated and shrunk within a few weeks. This is often possible with the use of over-the-counter medications and creams. In more severe cases, however, it may take longer for a hemorrhoid to completely shrink.

If you are concerned about how long it is taking for your hemorrhoid to completely shrink, it is important to speak to your doctor. They will be able to offer advice and guidance on the best course of treatment. Additionally, they will be able to monitor the progress of the hemorrhoid and offer reassurance if it is taking longer than expected to completely disappear.

The most important thing to remember when dealing with hemorrhoids is to keep the area clean. This means gently washing the area with warm water and avoiding any harsh cleansers. When drying, be sure to pat the area dry instead of rubbing. And, when using the restroom, be sure to wipe gently. If you experience any pain, bleeding, or itching, be sure to see your doctor, as these could be signs of a more serious problem.

Are Hemorrhoids More Common in Men than in Women?

Are hemorrhoids more common in men than in women? This is a question that has been asked by many people who suffer from this condition. The answer is not as simple as one might think.

There are many factors that contribute to the development of hemorrhoids. One of the most important factors is the amount of pressure that is placed on the veins in the anal region. This pressure can be caused by a variety of things, such as constipation, diarrhea, pregnancy, and obesity.

men tend to place more pressure on the veins in the anal region than women. This is due to a variety of factors, such as the fact that men tend to be larger than women, and they also have a greater amount of muscle mass.

This extra pressure can cause the veins to become engorged and eventually lead to the formation of hemorrhoids.

Another factor that contributes to the development of hemorrhoids is the amount of time that someone spends sitting. This is because sitting places extra pressure on the veins in the anal region. People who have sedentary jobs or who spend a lot of time sitting are at a higher risk for developing hemorrhoids.

There are a few risk factors that are more common in women than in men. These include pregnancy and giving birth. This is because the extra weight of the baby puts extra pressure on the veins in the anal region. Women who have had multiple pregnancies are even more at risk.

So, are hemorrhoids more common in men than in women? The answer is complicated. There are many factors that contribute to the development of hemorrhoids, and some of these factors are more common in men than in women. However, there are also some risk factors that are more common in women. So, it is impossible to say definitively whether or not men are more likely to develop hemorrhoids than women.

If you're dealing with hemorrhoids, you're not alone. Hemorrhoids are common, and they often occur with age. Luckily, there are many treatments available to help relieve the discomfort associated with hemorrhoids. If home remedies don't work, don't hesitate to see your doctor for other options.

What are prolapsed hemorrhoids?

Pregnancy, obesity, chronic constipation or diarrhea, anal intercourse, and aging all contribute to the development of hemorrhoids. Straining to poop can make existing hemorrhoids worse. Hemorrhoids are usually only treated if they are causing uncomfortable symptoms, such as itchiness, pain, or bleeding.

There are two types of hemorrhoids: internal and external hemorrhoids. Internal hemorrhoids are located inside of the rectum. External hemorrhoids are located under the skin around the anus.

Most hemorrhoids can be treated at home with over-the-countercreams, ointments, and pads. More severe hemorrhoids may require prescription medication or surgery.

Prolapsed hemorrhoids are a type of hemorrhoid that bulges out from the anus. Prolapsed hemorrhoids can be uncomfortable and painful. They can also be very dangerous if not treated immediately.

Prolapsed hemorrhoids happen when the tissue that supports the hemorrhoids weakens. This can be caused by pregnancy, obesity, chronic constipation or diarrhea, anal intercourse, and aging. Straining to poop can make existing hemorrhoids worse.

Prolapsed hemorrhoids can be very dangerous if not treated immediately. If the hemorrhoid bulges out too far, it can tear. This can cause bleeding and pain. If the hemorrhoid gets infected, it can cause a serious infection in the body.

Prolapsed hemorrhoids need to be treated by a doctor. If the hemorrhoid is not too severe, the doctor may be able to put it back in place. More severe prolapsed hemorrhoids may require surgery.

Hemorrhoids are a common and uncomfortable problem that can be effectively treated with home remedies, over-the-counter (OTC) medications, and surgery. With proper treatment, hemorrhoids usually go away within a few weeks. However, some people may experience recurrent hemorrhoids, which can be a sign of a more serious underlying condition. If home remedies and OTC medications don't improve hemorrhoids, or if they cause bleeding, contact your doctor.

Are Hemorrhoids a Disease?

Are hemorrhoids a disease? The answer isn't a simple one. Hemorrhoids can be a condition, a symptom of another problem, or even a side effect of certain medications.

Most people think of hemorrhoids as a condition caused by excessive straining during bowel movements. This straining can be a result of constipation, which is often caused by a diet low in fiber. Straining puts extra pressure on the veins in your rectum and anus, causing them to swell and bulge. This can cause bleeding, pain, and itching.

Hemorrhoids can also be a symptom of other problems. For example, they can be a sign of an intestinal blockage, inflammation, or infection. If you have hemorrhoids, it's important to see a doctor to rule out these other possibilities.

Finally, hemorrhoids can be a side effect of certain medications. These include prescription blood pressure medications and non-steroidal anti-inflammatory drugs (NSAIDs). If you take any of these medications and develop hemorrhoids, be sure to talk to your doctor. They may be able to switch you to a different medication.

In short, the answer to the question "are hemorrhoids a disease?" isn't a simple one. But understanding what hemorrhoids are and what causes them can help you find the best treatment for your particular situation.

There are many treatments for hemorrhoids, but the best way to avoid them is to prevent them. To do this, eat a high-fiber diet, drink plenty of water, and get regular exercise. If you already have hemorrhoids, there are a number of things you can do to relieve your symptoms and make them go away.

Do all prolapsed hemorrhoids need surgery?

A prolapsed hemorrhoid is a hemorrhoid that has enlarged and protrusions from the anal canal. not all prolapsed hemorrhoids will need surgery, however, depending on the severity of the prolapse.

Prolapsed hemorrhoids can be classified into three grades:

Grade I: The prolapse is internal and cannot be seen or felt outside the anal canal.

Grade II: The prolapse is external and can be seen or felt outside the anal canal, but it spontaneously returns inside the anal canal.

Grade III: The prolapse is external and can be seen or felt outside the anal canal, but it cannot be pushed back inside the anal canal.

Grade IV: The prolapse is external and can be seen or felt outside the anal canal, and it is accompanied by bleeding.

If your prolapsed hemorrhoid is grade I or II, you may be able to treat it with home remedies. If your prolapsed hemorrhoid is grade III or IV, you will likely need surgery to treat it.

Home remedies for prolapsed hemorrhoids include:

- eating a high-fiber diet

- drinking plenty of water

- taking over-the-counter (OTC) pain relievers

- applying OTC hemorrhoid creams or ointments

- using OTC suppositories for prolapsed hemorrhoids

- doing Gentle warm water baths

If home remedies don't work, you may need surgery to fix your prolapsed hemorrhoid. In some cases, you may need surgery if home remedies don't work and your prolapsed hemorrhoid is causing:

- severe pain

- bleeding

- fecal incontinence

There are a few different types of surgeries for prolapsed hemorrhoids. The type of surgery you have will depend on the severity of your prolapse.

Can you leave a prolapsed hemorrhoid untreated?

A prolapsed hemorrhoid is a hemorrhoid that has protruded from the anus and has blood vessels and tissue around it. When left untreated, prolapsed hemorrhoids can strangulate, meaning the blood supply is cut off, and the tissue around the hemorrhoid dies. This can cause severe pain and, in some cases, infection. If you have a prolapsed hemorrhoid, it is important to see a doctor as soon as possible to have it treated.

Hemorrhoids are a common problem that can be painful and uncomfortable. However, there are many treatments available that can help relieve the symptoms. With proper treatment, most people with hemorrhoids can get relief from their symptoms and live a normal life.

Bleeding from a Popped Hemorrhoid ?

A popped hemorrhoid can bleed for a while. This usually happens when the hemorrhoid becomes engorged with blood and then ruptures. The blood can sometimes be bright red, and it can drip or even gush out of the anus. It can be frightening to see this happen, but it is not usually a sign of anything serious.

If a hemorrhoid pops, it will often bleed for a few minutes before stopping. If the bleeding does not stop or if it is severe, then it is important to see a doctor. There is a small chance that a hemorrhoid that bleeds a lot can be a sign of something more serious, such as colon cancer. However, this is very rare.

There are a few things that you can do to help stop the bleeding from a popped hemorrhoid. First, try to apply pressure to the area with a clean cloth. This will help to stop the bleeding. Second, try to avoid straining or sitting for long periods of time. This can make the hemorrhoid bleed more. Finally, try to eat a high-fiber diet and drink plenty of fluids. This will help to soften your stool and make it easier to pass.

Hemorrhoids are a common affliction that can cause a great deal of pain and discomfort. Although they can be a nuisance, they are usually not a serious condition and can be treated with over-the-counter medication and home remedies. In severe cases, hemorrhoids may require medical treatment. If you are experiencing pain or bleeding, be sure to see your doctor to rule out any other potential causes.

Can you get rid of prolapsed hemorrhoids on your own?

Hemorrhoids are a sensitive subject for many people who suffer from them. They can be both painful and itchy, and can make everyday activities quite difficult. Many people with hemorrhoids often wonder if there is anything they can do to get rid of them.

There are a few different types of hemorrhoids, but the most common are internal hemorrhoids. These are located inside the rectum and are often not visible. Prolapsed hemorrhoids are a type of internal hemorrhoid that bulges out from the anal opening. External hemorrhoids are located outside of the anal opening and are often visible.

There are a few different ways to treat hemorrhoids, but not all of them are effective for everyone. Some people may be able to get rid of their prolapsed hemorrhoids on their own, but others may need medical intervention.

If you are able to get rid of your prolapsed hemorrhoids on your own, there are a few things you can do to help make the process easier. First, you will want to make sure that you are drinking plenty of water. This will help to keep your stool soft, which will make it easier to pass. You will also want to add more fiber to your diet. This can be done by eating more fruits and vegetables, or by taking a fiber supplement.

There are a few over-the-counter treatments that you can try, but it is important to talk to your doctor before using any of them. These treatments can help to shrink the hemorrhoids, but they will not get rid of them completely. If you are not able to get rid of your prolapsed hemorrhoids on your own, or if your symptoms are severe, you may need to have them surgically removed.

Talk to your doctor about your options for getting rid of prolapsed hemorrhoids. They will be able to tell you what the best course of treatment is for your individual situation.

Should I worry about a prolapsed hemorrhoid?

A prolapsed hemorrhoid is a hemorrhoid that has fallen down from the anal canal. It can be quite painful, especially if it gets trapped between the buttocks. If you have a prolapsed hemorrhoid, you should see a doctor to have it treated.

To conclude, hemorrhoids are a common and often painful condition that can be caused by a variety of things, including constipation, pregnancy, and obesity. There are a number of treatments available, both home remedies and medical procedures, so it is important to talk to your doctor to find the best course of treatment for you.

T

he difference between a hemorrhoid and a prolapse

A hemorrhoid is an enlarged vein in the anus or lower rectum. A prolapse occurs when the rectum or anal canal becomes displaced and comes out through the anus. The main difference between hemorrhoids and prolapse is that hemorrhoids are usually not painful, while prolapse often is. prolapse can also lead to more serious complications, such as incontinence or intestinal blockage.

While hemorrhoids can be painful, they are usually not serious. Hemorrhoids may clear up on their own after a few days, and many people who have them don't even know they have them. However, if hemorrhoids bleed a lot, cause pain, or make it difficult to pass stool, you should see a doctor.

Medical treatment for hemorrhoids include:

Medical treatment for hemorrhoids often includes a combination of lifestyle changes, over the counter medication, and prescription medication.

If your hemorrhoids are mild, you may be able to treat them with lifestyle changes, like eating more fiber, drinking more water, and exercising. You can also try over-the-counter topical cream or ointments.

If your hemorrhoids are more severe, your doctor may prescribe oral medication or a pill that you can insert into your rectum. If your hemorrhoids are very severe, you may need to have surgery.

If you have hemorrhoids, you're not alone. Hemorrhoids are common and usually not too serious. They can often be treated with home remedies, and you may not need to see a doctor. But some types of hemorrhoids can cause bleeding that can be dangerous. If your hemorrhoids bleed a lot, see a doctor. Also, see a doctor if hemorrhoids don't go away, even with home treatment.

Inflamed blood vessels

Inflamed blood vessels can cause a lot of discomfort and pain. Hemorrhoids are one type of inflamed blood vessel. Hemorrhoids are when the veins around your anus or in your lower rectum become swollen and inflamed. This can happen after you have a baby, from straining during a bowel movement, or from sitting for a long time on the toilet. Hemorrhoids can be internal, which means they are inside your rectum, or they can be external, which means they are under the skin around your anus.

If you have hemorrhoids, you may notice that you bleed when you have a bowel movement. You may also see blood on the toilet paper or in the toilet bowl. Hemorrhoids can be uncomfortable, and you may feel itchiness or pain around your anus. If a hemorrhoid pops out of your anus, it can be very painful.

There are many things you can do to ease the discomfort and pain of hemorrhoids. Soak in a warm bath for 20 minutes a day. This will help to reduce inflammation. Apply a hemorrhoid cream or ointment to the area to ease itchiness and pain. Place a cold pack on the area for a few minutes to numb the pain. If your hemorrhoids are very large and painful, you may need to see a doctor to have them removed.

There are many different ways to treat hemorrhoids, depending on the severity of the condition. In most cases, however, hemorrhoids can be treated at home with over-the-counter medications, Dorsey says. If symptoms persist or appear more than once per week, however, it's time to see a doctor for evaluation and possible treatment with prescription-strength medications or other procedures.

* 9 7 8 1 7 7 6 9 6 9 6 2 3 *
SD - #0030 - 140926 - C0 - 229/152/15 - PB - 9781776969623 - Matt Lamination